*Tracie*

# ROSA'S CHOICE

## HEALING THE WOUNDS OF THE MOTHER

A journey into the world of the spirit baby
and how we can build a New Earth, together.

*With love and blessings*

Debra Kilby

*Debra Yxxx*

ISBN:

Paperback: 978-1-913590-17-8

Ebook: 978-1-913590-18-5


Cover design by Lynda Mangoro, Creative Genie.


The Unbound Press

www.theunboundpress.com

**Hey unbound one!**

Welcome to this magical book brought to you by The Unbound Press.

At The Unbound Press we believe that when women write freely from the fullest expression of who they are, it can't help but activate a feeling of deep connection and transformation in others. When we come together, we become more and we're changing the world, one book at a time!

This book has been carefully crafted by both the author and publisher with the intention of inspiring you to move ever more deeply into who you truly are.

We hope that this book helps you to connect with your Unbound Self and that you feel called to pass it on to others who want to live a more fully expressed life.

With much love,

*Nicola Humber*

Founder of The Unbound Press

www.theunboundpress.com

This book is dedicated to Rosa, to my own and all spirit babies who offer their love in service to waking us up as individuals and all humanity.

It's dedicated to all women who are rising through their pain into their innate loving Truth and wisdom. And the men that love, recognise, and encourage us all to step into our true power.

A huge thank you to my tribe of 'dragons', you know who you are! My soul sisters and friends who have seen me through the doubts, the highs and the lows of the birthing of this book. Hazel Boylan for her patience and lovingly running her expert editing eye over my words. My best friend Sam Flambard, Karen Goodson and Renira Barclay for their reassurance, support and time in reading my words pre-publishing.

And of course, last but not least, my husband Lee, my boys Max and Samuel, who keep me grounded, surrounded in love, laughter, belief and much, much more.

I wish for this book to be a blessing in your own awakening and deeper connection to yourself and the other realms, helping to transform the world to bring about a New Earth.

Together, we rise. And so it is.

With love,

Debra

# Contents

## Part ONE

## Part TWO

## Part THREE

# Part ONE

# Rosa's Message from the Spirit Baby Realm for Humanity

So here is where we start and here is where we end, for there really is no end or beginning of this story. It is just the moment that I have chosen to allow access to the realm of spirit and the true life pictures our babies gift us with.

So listen well, you women of light who are drawn to this book, for in it lies some mysteries to the Universe, and you are all the key.

There comes a time in our lives when a choice has to be made. A choice based on love and a choice based on truth. We cannot live in the darkness for much longer or it will overwhelm each and every one of us. It is time for the light – a light that is spreading far and wide.

Do not fear if you are chosen for this path, for it is one you had already chosen many lifetimes ago. Whether that be as a mum or a grandmother, a sister, an aunty, or a cherished friend, or one who serves and supports these women in the highest of ways, this book will reach into your heart and soul and you will know your path in this New Earth.

For I am Rosa, and I am here to spread the light. And with your help, we can do so.

Do not fret if your baby has not yet appeared. Do not fret if your baby has disappeared from view. Because they are all here. They are all here and waiting for you to accept their mission as carriers of light – into the wombs of women who are the holders of light.

Are you one of the holders of light? If you are reading this you surely are. If you doubt your ability to do this, then do not doubt, for we are all here by your side. It is this doubt, fear, and lack that keep us, your spirit babies, from coming to you. For the circumstances of our birth must be of the light. Of a moment where our circumstances allow us to enter, knowing our own missions are fully supported and upheld by the ones we choose.

So clear your doubt, your fear and unworthiness, for we are here, and we will come when you do so, our very special women of the light who have led the way.

There is no time for us to come into darkness and work through it. Many of us have already been there and done that and now we only wish to shed light from the very beginning.

For that, we need our special souls on earth to pave the way so the path is clear and we are not held up by judgement or self-loathing or impossibility. For everything is possible and everything is very much real.

Find your path, find yourself and you will find us. Don't be distressed if this seems like a huge task, it is not, not in the bigger sense of the world. For all your heartaches and lessons have brought you to this place and the light is coming to help you realise this. To shine a light on your experiences so far, in order that you can step into your role as a mother of the New Earth.

Do not be daunted by your task. All will be made clear to you on connection with your baby's soul. These baby souls are ready and waiting for you in masses that have yet to be seen in the world.

The truth is that you are all Mother Marys – all of you who are on this mission – in the sense that Mother Mary is known for giving birth to the light.

It is not that you will be giving birth to Jesus Christ; you will be giving birth to your own baby soul on a much higher level, cleansed and cleared of all past lives, of all layers that may hold it back from being love and bringing joy to the world in its purest forms.

The Mother Mary in each of you is essentially the carrier of these special souls. Those of you who have learnt your own lessons, have cleared your own disbeliefs and are ready to welcome in the souls of light that will change the world.

It really is no biggie – they are still your babies. They will still need love and care and bring with them the frustration and heartache that come with babies. The difference is that they have chosen you to hold and guide them in their own specialness. Understand deeply where they have come from and why they are here, so that you can serve their best interests and allow them fully to embrace the changes they are here to bring.

Much is wrong with your world and how you see children. How you stifle their souls to fit in with what is. These new souls will not be stifled, nor will they adhere to the rules your society has set.

In every other way, they are the same as all baby souls, the difference is they will awaken the world with their light, as you, as their chosen ones, allow their light to shine and in the fullest and brightest of ways.

## They are here – are you?

If you are ready, then read on. Read these words of wisdom from other realms to form a true picture of your world and ours. There is nothing to fear for there is only love. You are being asked, being called upon, to let this love in once and for all.

You bravest and kindest souls, you women of the world, it is time to rise, and rise you will, for that is the way it is meant to be. No more the darkness that took this power from you, no more is the mindset that love is weakness and hope a pointless exercise.

No more the woes and the battles, the greed and the power and all the distortions this brings. It is time for women; it is time for the sacred feminine. Your men are part of this – the real men who see the power of women and embrace it and do not diminish it through their own lens of fear.

There are many parents sought by the world today, for it is time, it is coming, and it is written in the stars. Rise, dear women, and allow the power you feel inside to bubble up to the surface and shine.

Shine so brightly it will change the outlook of the world and all its people. Be ready, be willing, be open, for all is coming and all is possible.

# Introduction

On 26 November 2010, when I was sixteen weeks pregnant, I had a call from the hospital. It was two days before my son Max's third birthday. This was the fourth time I had become pregnant since my husband and I had been blessed with Max in 2007. Between 2007 and 2009 we lived through three miscarriages. Surely this one would be okay, we hoped.

Being pregnant with Max was easy, fun, and exciting, but his birth was not what I had expected. The shock and fear I experienced affected how I felt about being a mum.

However, nine months into motherhood, and with the traumas nicely buried, we fell pregnant again. This baby news was something of a surprise, but welcomed, and we felt we could conquer all practicalities – and wasn't it great that they would be so close in age?

However, a week before the twelve-week scan, I started to bleed. The bleeding didn't stop and eventually I had to be rushed to hospital. That was my first experience of miscarriage and the overwhelming helplessness and loss of my little one. My failure.

I picked myself up relatively quickly, quoting all sorts of statistics at myself about how one in four women lose their babies and how, generations before pregnancy testing, women didn't even know they were pregnant and so miscarriage was normal and you just got on with life. I didn't ask for help and I didn't allow myself the time or the space to grieve and acknowledge my hurt and disappointment.

Over the next two years, I conceived easily but they didn't stay longer than eight and twelve weeks. By this time my heart had closed, but I wasn't aware of the effect of all this loss, because I didn't allow myself to feel it.

And then along came Rosa.

I was both excited and terrified of how this pregnancy would go. I did have some bleeding at nine weeks and rushed to the hospital for a scan. Thank goodness all was well with her little heart beating away. The bleeding stopped.

But I had the strangest experience one night when I was reading in bed. I heard the words come from outside of myself: "Mummy, I'm sick". I told my husband and we put it down to the obvious fear I was experiencing because of our last three miscarriages. But somehow I knew – despite all the scans, including the twelve-week scan – that something was very wrong.

I am now aware that I am an intuitive with the ability to tune into the energies of people here and in spirit, and in particular spirit babies. In fact, my son, Max, had introduced himself at around eight weeks into the pregnancy with, "Hi Mum, my name's Jack". Obviously, we didn't go with the name, and it took the surprise out of the gender, but those whom I told about this found it fascinating and amusing and not surprising at all. Because us mums know deep down we can connect with our babies, even if we choose not to fully embrace this.

But I didn't fully understand that back then. Now when I think of Rosa's little words coming to me, gently preparing me, I hold onto that connection we so clearly had. That we all have as mums.

After a number of incidents, my knowing that something was wrong was finally confirmed. The hospital phoned me with the results of the tests. Rosa wasn't developing as she should be due to genetic complications. She was diagnosed with Down Syndrome and I was told she was unlikely to make it to full term, and if she did, it was uncertain what quality of life she would enjoy.

My heart and my world broke. How could this possibly be happening to me? What had I ever done to deserve this pain? Now I know many families with children who are not 'perfect' in society's eyes, but who, of course, are utterly perfect in every single way. And they are in this world, as we all are, to create their own special path.

But I did not fully see this at that time. I didn't know about souls and soul plans and choices and life paths. I only saw what my own life experiences and conditioning told me.

And so this is where I am choosing to start our story. And even as I sit here writing, despite knowing what I know now, it is still with a tiny sense of disbelief and some trepidation at what I am about to share. But also in the absolute knowing that I am ready to write it, people are ready to read it, and it is one hundred percent the right thing to do.

I also know at the very core of my being that writing and saying the following statement is what I believe in the depths of my soul. This declaration may be shocking or downright odd to some of you, but stay with me – I felt the same when I first heard these words come out of my own mouth.

Saying a heartbreaking hello and goodbye to my daughter, Rosa, before twenty weeks of pregnancy had passed, was the greatest challenge and greatest gift I have ever received.

Of course, at the time this was as far from what I was feeling as you can possibly imagine. Because I didn't lose Rosa because of some dreadful accident, or inexplicable miscarriage. I chose to release her. And it was one of the hardest decisions I have ever had to make or wish to make ever again.

Not only would I have had to potentially endure the loss of yet another much-wanted baby, and this time at a stage where I would have to give birth, but I would also have had to choose whether to stay with it and see if she survived. And if she survived, how long might that be for? What would her life be like? What would our life be like? I'd just turned forty and what if she did survive but needed looking after – as we got older, would that eventually fall to Max and entirely dictate the path of his life? How would we cope?

The miscarriages were out of my control. This was a whole other level. I had to make a choice, together with my husband – but ultimately it felt like mine. I can safely say from that moment on I don't believe I was present in this world.

I can barely remember the next few days. When the midwife gave me the pill that would end Rosa's life, I wanted to throw up, then curl into a ball and die with her. But life has a way of keeping you going in some form and for me, that was our beautiful Max and the love of my husband, Lee.

The birth is a blur but I can recall the physical and emotional pain as my husband and I said hello and goodbye to her. We knew then it was a girl.

I shut down then. I didn't want to know. I told myself it was just something that happened and to get on with it. But I wasn't really there. The hospital said they arranged funerals for babies and my immediate reaction was no – she wasn't a baby. It's shocking how much I tried to deny this experience. But we don't act sanely in these moments.

Eventually, I started to wonder more about Rosa. Why, and why me? Where is she? Who is she? And how am I ever going to come through this? With the most amazing support from the charity ARC – Antenatal Results and Choices – eventually, we chose to go ahead with the funeral. It was the most beautiful, poignant moment and the start of my healing.

As I was sitting in the garden afterwards, I allowed myself to see how I was truly feeling for the first time since my first miscarriage. It wasn't pretty! The loss, the sense of being a victim, being a failure, being undeserving of any joy, being a terrible if not evil person.

The deep shame about the choice I'd made was so intense I hadn't told anyone except close family and a handful of friends. I don't know what my work colleagues thought of me at the time. All but three of them had no clue what was going on for me. I'm not tied to any religion, but I was working for a Catholic humanitarian organisation at the time – in my mind if they found out what I'd done I would lose my job. Such was the intensity of my shame.

Most of all, however, I felt overwhelming bitterness. I'd see a pregnant woman and feel a glimpse of joy. I'd then really try to feel happy for her and all I came back to was: but what about me? Why them and not me? This was the feeling I loathed the most as it felt against my very nature. "This is not me," I thought.

And then it struck me. Who is this me who doesn't want to be bitter and angry and sad and closed off? It was then I went on a journey to find that me, that part of me that wasn't all these negative emotions created by the layers of life, but the real me. The me that was loving and happy and adventurous and believed in miracles and possibilities.

And this is why I am forever grateful to our beautiful Rosa. By giving away love through the choice I made, she gave me back myself. And my whole world has changed beyond my imagination.

At 42, I gave birth happily and easily to another gorgeous boy, Samuel. I thought I might need counselling throughout the pregnancy, but I didn't. I just knew deep down that all was well. By addressing and clearing my experiences through energy-healing practices, connecting with this beautiful soul we now know as Samuel before he even arrived, and ultimately forgiving myself, I knew he was meant to be. He is my miracle. The fact is, we are all miracles.

Ultimately, I chose love. The love of letting go. The love of myself and all the things that wouldn't come to pass with Rosa physically in our lives. And the love of Rosa and her life. A choice of love which was to be more profound than I ever imagined at that time.

It is now my utmost passion and mission to guide women to their own knowing and empowerment. To help women realise that they do not need to be defined by their experience – no matter how bad they feel about it, or themselves – or to feel stuck in their emotions. There are many gentle and beautiful ways to feel whole and at peace with yourself and your life.

Through the course of my healing and deeper understanding of life before life, and life after death, I now choose the word 'releasing' rather than use the word 'termination'. As you read through Rosa's messages, and the one on termination in particular, you'll realise that life cannot be terminated.

Since releasing Rosa, I have discovered, and am still discovering, there is always a much, much bigger and more magnificent picture behind the journey to motherhood; a whole other world and reason behind baby loss and struggling to conceive. My wish is that by the end of this book, particularly Part 1, you will begin to see a chink of light at the end of the tunnel you may be in.

## Your soul journey

Your challenging journey to motherhood is not separate from your soul journey – it is your soul journey; pushing you to dig deep inside yourself, to truly know yourself and break free of this lifetime's, and ancient lifetimes', patterns of being powerless, being less than, not knowing you are a creator. The challenge of your journey is gifting you with the opportunity to know yourself on a deeply profound level as a person and as a portal so loving, so courageous, so powerful that you are able to invite, hold, and transform energy into form, and to birth new life, new consciousness, into the world.

You need you. Your babies need you. And the earth needs you to know just how incredible, magical, and miraculous you are. You don't need to get your head around all the messages in this book until you want to or need to. You don't need to do anything other than allow yourself the opportunity to unravel all that life has shown you and find the truth of you within it. Not mine, not Rosa's, not anyone else's – purely yours, as the beautiful soul you are on the unique journey you're on.

My heartfelt wish is that through the pain you come to joy, that you hold your babies in your arms, or meet them in spirit and understand your why.

# The New Earth, the Mother Wound and a Potential Future

In Part 1 of this book, you'll be introduced to concepts around the New Earth, the mother wound, and – setting the scene for the rest of this book – where this is taking us for the future of yourself, your children and all of us. I'll share who am I to write this book and why am I doing it, who Rosa is, and why she is sharing her messages.

We'll be exploring the many forms of baby loss including miscarriage, still birth and termination. And why women may be struggling to conceive from the perspective of the spirit babies. Why they choose not to stay, or why they choose to wait to arrive. We'll look at what's in the way of conceiving and highlight areas of healing for you, the individual. Also covered are the various ways your baby chooses to arrive, whether naturally or through IVF, egg donation, or adoption. Part 1 is all about the beautiful dance you are on with your baby, leading to insight into where this is all heading in terms of a New Earth, a new way of being and freedom.

This book is essentially about the energy of creation. That is who we are, our essence. We are all created, creative, and therefore, creation; it's what we're here for – to create. We create in every moment. Whether that be your life or a new life. All of which not only affects you but the collective.

What us courageous women and men are doing here through our challenging journeys to motherhood, to parenthood, is blatantly showing the world that something is very wrong, something is out of balance. If we are not creating and creative, this is against the natural law of who we are. The more out of balance this energy of creation is, the more out of balance we are in terms of being creative, the more the earth becomes out of balance. We are all here to find balance within ourselves in order to bring balance, restore balance in the world, and, yes, the Universe.

# Building a New Earth

In 2010, I never imagined I would be writing a book, let alone one that would be written in collaboration with the spirit baby and soul mentor I call Rosa. But here we are.

I have read the message from Rosa that opens this book many times, but I only now understand the layers of information that it and the others throughout this book contain.

It is only through writing this book (guided, pushed, nudged, kicked even by spirit to do so) that – just when I think I have the structure and the information down – new and more mind-blowing information comes through.

I believe we are only shown what we are ready and able to understand. If we knew it all in one go it would blow our minds or lead us to dismiss it, or ridicule it even, as many seers and prophets have been. We have to be ready to hear it. And if you have come by this book, then you are ready to hear it and maybe, hopefully, feel supported enough to step up into the role you came here for. Your role in building, birthing, a New Earth.

I was shown a glimpse of this New Earth one day and it is almost impossible to describe the feeling of it. I was running one of my courses – From Here to Maternity: 7 Steps to Meeting Your Baby – and we'd just completed the Kundalini yoga class for opening the third eye. I was relaxing in meditation, guided by my yoga teacher for this course, Linda Martin, when a new spirit guide showed up. He was of Aboriginal descent and he asked me to walk with him over the brow of a hill. At the top, I saw the most magnificent sunrise, huge and glowing with reds, oranges and yellows. "A New Dawn", he said.

I was silenced by the beauty of it. A few weeks later I was being nudged to connect with my new guide again. I asked him how I could help. Again, it is almost impossible to describe – stay with me here. It was as if Mother Earth came inside my body so I could see through her eyes. I moved through the sunrise of the New Dawn to see and feel how she saw herself. Magnificent barely covers it. So much beauty, lush and abundant, and a feeling of such peace and love. For me, it felt like freedom – my version of Eden. I saw the children of the New Earth then, busy playing and learning in their forest schools, free. Life, play, learning, medicine, all provided for by the earth. There was technology but not as we know it.

I realised that the earth already saw herself as the New Earth, it's already here, it already is. Whenever we all choose to see it or believe it's possible for it to be a physical reality beyond the veils of pain, structure, and fear. The more people who are able to envisage or feel this energy, the closer it becomes to reality. The New Earth children are of this energy and are bringing this vision of unity and cooperation, playfulness and freedom with them to help us all move towards it. If we wish to, of course.

My new course was then born, in that moment as I was asked to guide women to reactivate/remember this New Earth, New Dawn energy in their wombs: Sacred Conception. A New Dawn – Birthing the Children of the New Earth. (You can find out more about this course in the notes at the back of this book.)

A new dawn is upon us. Mother Earth needs us, needs you, to begin to see yourself and the world in a different way, a more loving and connected way; one of self-belief, your Divine right as a sovereign being, a return to feeling whole, worthy, a life of equality and self-love. Just as the earth called you, the earth is calling your baby to her in order to literally bring heaven down to earth; to create beautiful transformation in the way the world works, how we treat ourselves, each other and the earth.

*"For a new dawn to be conceived and birthed, there has to be a new way of conceiving and birthing."*

When I think about this vision in terms of the energy system known as the chakras, we rest and grow in the womb, the physical place closest to the sacral chakra but also the solar plexus and root chakra. At birth, our crown chakra, our connection to Source, meets the root chakra of our mothers. Imagine this experience if there is fear, insecurity, and shame held in the root. Does this create an early block in our connection to ourselves and our remembrance of who we are? Now imagine being birthed through an energy of safety, love, and connection to earth and body. I wonder, as we heal the pain so often held in our lower three chakras, how much less of an impact this would have on distorting our connection to ourselves and Source. A vision the spirit babies show me is an airplane coming into land: one with a runway littered with debris that makes the landing a little more precarious and therefore a less safe feeling of arrival; and another a runway that is clear. We're all being asked to clear our runways as much as possible. For those of you wishing to conceive, with a clearer runway the babies and future babies would  arrive more 'awake' to who they are because they haven't had to pass through quite so much density. The colours of A New Dawn sunrise are the same colours as the lower three chakras. Just a thought! This is not to pile on even more guilt or blame by the way, we all carry blocks in some form from this lifetime, past and ancestral hurts and traumas. Being aware of this and bringing awareness to them for healing is a step to freeing yourself and any future babies.

There's so much going on in our world now at the time of writing in 2020 that looks and feels the exact opposite of this New Earth vision. In moments where I feel hopeless or helpless because of what's going on, I remind myself of the overwhelming energy of love I felt in this New Earth vision. If this energy is here and accessible to us all, then I know everything really will be okay.

Rosa's message below offers the spiritual perspective of the New Earth, and how we came to forget it in the first place.

**What is the New Earth? Let Rosa describe it:**

> This earth that you all talk about is not in fact a New Earth but an old earth, an original earth, the earth it has always been. And yet, much like you, slightly damaged, bruised, lost and confused as to why anyone would want to destroy her in the first place. For all the earth was and still is, is love. Just like you.

Yet there were some who chose to destroy this earth, plunder it, and damage it. Why? Why destroy the very thing that gave them life? Gave them life in the form of love, the force that is love, unconditional love.

You could argue that some were envious of the light, the love that came from it – the life that came from it. They too wanted to be the ones who could create life.

They wished to be the womb and the birther and the creator of life, and they were jealous. They were jealous because they were lacking, lacking in this most creative of life force-giving energies, little understanding that they were indeed the other very much needed half to that creation. But no, they wanted it all.

They wanted to be the creators, the lovers, the birthers, and the birthed. And they could not bear that some could do things and create miracles that they could not. So they started to suppress these miracles. And they started to make it a bad thing to bleed; a bad thing to die.

They made everything a 'bad' thing and so people felt they only had one way to turn – and that was bad. And yet, thankfully, there were some among us who were so good, so good they knew the way, they knew the light, and if only we all followed them we would be safe, we would be saved, we would be 'seen' to be good, even if we didn't feel good on the inside.

Here is where our dilemma and conflict arose. For how could this be good, when it felt bad being told how we 'should' be? And what did it matter to be seen to be good, if those being seen to be good were bad? Those who said they were good and to follow their way, even if we felt them to be bad?

But if we did not 'see' their goodness, then were we not bad? Were we not under threat of being bad? And if we could see the bad in the good and the good in the bad – then how were we ever to come to a place of alignment? A place of agreement, a place of love, of understanding and compassion?

The truth is, we no longer knew ourselves. We no longer knew who we were as a 'whole' person of both the good and the bad and the in-between and the all and everything of the all and everything. Our sense of self was questioned, judged, and taken apart. It came that we eventually accepted we were all okay with this not knowing of who we were. We all knew we didn't know who we were and therefore understood ourselves and each other.

Yet here we are in a time where we are talking about a New Earth, a new way of being. In fact, all we are doing is being returned, returning to our original selves. Returning to the light of which we are and not the dark of which we have been told to be.

There is no more of this, good and bad, but only the compassion, love, and understanding for the many great things that have inspired and transpired to the bringing back of the light, the bringing back of the Divine Feminine of which we are all a part. The bringing back of birth as a celebration and a miracle of women, with the love or the seed of a man to bring about the wholeness that is needed in order for a divine child to be born.

And so, my dear, all we are doing is returning to the light and the knowledge that lies there, that we are all indeed One. That we all have a role to play in building that light and no one or no thing can or needs to be coerced for any more time.

And this is the way it was and this is the way it will be.

And so it is.

# What is Rosa saying?

Each of Rosa's messages contain layers of information, another one being revealed each time you are ready to see it. Whatever layer of understanding you receive from them, please know reading the words themselves, and being with this book, will be healing. Rosa is planting beautiful seeds for growth. It's entirely up to you if you accept them.

My current reading of her messages is that we were once whole, felt wholeness and oneness with ourselves, others, and the earth, and at some point in time, this was fractured. We became confused, separate and lost our sense of self. The earth gave, just as women, the feminine, the mother did, from a place of love but this was corrupted and turned into a 'bad' thing. Controlled and taken from, rather than free and given and giving to.

We as women are being asked to lift off our own personal layers of blame, shame, unworthiness, and fear that we've carried for centuries. To question whether what we believe is our truth or someone else's, and heal the wounds of the feminine, the wounds of the mother, in order to shine our light ever more brightly. This book is focused on women but it's the same for men, the other vital half of creation, to courageously look within.

As each individual does this, we heal not only ourselves, but all mothers right back to the original mother wound of the Divine Feminine, the Divine Mother, and ultimately, Mother Earth herself, if not indeed the Universe. Yes, you are that powerful and special! When we've lifted these wounds out of our physical and energy bodies, the babies have a much clearer runway to arrive on. One with less clutter and debris to potentially pick up or run into along the way. With these wounds no longer present, the children of the light who are already here, or who are waiting to be born, arrive in a New World, a New Earth, a new freedom in which they can create a very different way of life and being than we are currently seeing.

A way of life that is no longer driven by patriarchal power, greed, and ego, that for eons have supressed the feminine and abused the earth. A time when they, when all of us, will no longer feel under such pressure to go along with those in positions of power in various structures and institutions, who claim they hold the truth or hold the light and therefore are the rightful leaders. Instead, we will begin to see the Truth and the light and the power of ourselves. These children will see and create a New Earth because they are not carrying ancient wounds which have been passed from mother to mother to mother.

# What is the mother wound?

Why is it present and why is it so important to heal? When I received the inspiration for this book, in one big boom of a download one night, all I knew was that I wanted to write a book that would comfort and support women on their journeys to motherhood.

The mother wound, as I saw it back in 2016, was the deep, inexplicable hurt that comes from desperately wanting a baby and it not happening, or the hurt that comes through baby loss or birth trauma. I was very much focused on the lack of emotional support available to women at all stages of their motherhood journey and into parenthood, and wanted to fill that gap through my energy healing work and my writing of this book, Rosa's Choice.

The first part is the book that I wanted to write, the book that first came to me and is very much focused on you, the individual, finding ways to move through and forward on your journey with knowledge and insight from the spirit baby realm.

As I progressed in my own healing, experience and knowledge, this limited awareness of the mother wound grew exponentially for me, and I began to realise just how deep and how far back it goes, how many layers there are beyond what we experience as individuals. And then Part 2 and Part 3 of this book came into being. That is, the bigger picture.

In psychological terms, the mother wound is defined as your mother not being emotionally attuned and available to you as a child – often a repetition of your own mother's mother wound – lack of adequate, good-enough mothering, or emotional absence. Your mother not fulfilling your needs.

We are conscious beings in this lifetime from the moment of conception. It is not just genes that are passed down the ancestral line but also – as the study of epigenetics shows us – patterns of behaviour and beliefs, as well as traumas.

It's easy to interpret this as all the women's fault – and, goodness, don't a lot of us take that on board! It can stop here. It can stop with you. Enough. For me, it reminds me of the biblical notion that women are the cause of the downfall of 'Man' and therefore we have to spend our lives making up for it. This book will show you other perspectives and help guide you to a new awareness, new knowledge, and your own truth.

Let's move out of the blame game and explore what's really going on. Why is the pain there in the first place? What caused the original wound?

## Women are from Venus, men are from Mars

When I talk about masculine and feminine energies it's important to know this is not about gender. You have likely lived lifetimes as a male as well as a female. All of us hold both the masculine and feminine aspects – they are energies. One of the Universal Laws is the Law of Gender. It refers to the fact that there are two major types of energy. You can think of them as masculine and feminine, or yin and yang. We all contain a certain amount of both and must find a way to achieve a balance between the two if we are to live authentically and happily; to become co-creators.

Masculine energy is generally more associated with competition, results-based action and logic, the provider and protector, the survival-of-the-fittest type of energy. Feminine energy is associated with cooperation, relationship, nurturing, loving and deep. If you look at your life, you'll see from which of these areas you operate.

The healthiest trick overall is to find ways of integrating both the masculine and feminine energies within you to bring balance within yourself. Drawing on your feminine side for inspiration, to create and nurture your ideas from a place of love, drawing on your masculine to take action, and on both to bring your idea and creation into being.

The mother wound as I see it now, from a much wider perspective, began the moment the imbalance between the masculine and feminine shifted too far in favour of the masculine. As Rosa describes in her New Earth message above, and in many throughout this book, the moment the masculine felt unnerved and in so much fear of the power of the feminine which created through love – to feel the need to have power over it. This includes Mother Earth. The moment or series of moments the masculine felt the only way to feel safe, important, and of consequence to life, was to control it. The energy of fear has a way of making us want to control situations and people, as you've no doubt experienced yourself.

The mother wound is therefore ancient and deep. A deep wound coming from the beginnings of our patriarchal society in which women's power to love and create was punished, ridiculed, and controlled. Women's ability to create was slowly and subversively, or overtly, made to seem the opposite of special, the opposite of a gift, the opposite of a miracle, and therefore dirty and in need of controlling. You can see in our history how the Church, for example, has played a role in dismissing the feminine, at best, and corrupting the truth of the feminine for their own agenda, at worst.

Women, for eons of time, have been conditioned and, in most cases, have taken on board the belief that they are less than; that there is something wrong about them. This ingrained conditioning, essentially an aspect of 'I'm not good enough', has been passed down through generation upon generation of women.

Unconsciously, we've been left with this deep sense of guilt at having done something wrong, or that there is something wrong with us, purely by the fact of being female and being able to do what we do. We can then feel we're on a treadmill of constantly trying to make up for our 'wrongness' by pleasing everybody else, sacrificing ourselves for others' happiness to prove that we're not wrong or bad after all.

This is a big message to take on board and I hope I'm explaining it clearly because it is hard to find the words to describe an intangible energy and moment in time that may have no relevance to your life now. But through the messages from Rosa and my own and others' intuitive insights, it's basically saying that who we are now, what we are experiencing, and what women, in particular, have experienced for generations, goes back to a wound so ancient we can barely comprehend it.

We all carry this original mother wound. Our role, beautiful women, is to take responsibility for healing our own wounds. By so doing, you play your role in healing the original mother wound. Once released of this burden, you also free your ancestors and leave your daughters and sons, and future daughters and sons, with a legacy of freedom. Freedom to be themselves and express themselves in the world in a way that has not been possible since the times of the fabled lost civilisations of Lemuria and Atlantis where Oneness and cooperation were the experience.

When this wound is no longer present, the New Earth souls won't be looking at the world through the lens of patriarchy and all its traits and controls. Instead, they will have a clear vision, unclouded by the beliefs, patterns and programmes we see playing out today and which have played out across eons. They will come into a world where there is more balance. They will come into a world of love.

## Who is sacrificing themselves and why?

I so often hear mums saying, 'I've had to sacrifice so much for my children'. I even felt this myself when I became a mum – a disturbing collapse of my sense of self and identity. A grieving for who I thought I was and what my life was about. What I didn't realise then was that I hadn't lost my sense of self, because I had no idea who my real self was at that time. My identity was a total falsehood of conditioning and life experiences. It was a good identity, but it wasn't fully me.

When our desire to create life is compromised in some way, or when we prepare to become mums, and certainly when we become one, the subconscious mind opens up like a Pandora's box of emotions and beliefs that have been nicely hidden away from the moment of our own conception and beyond. Trying to become a mum, or losing a baby, or becoming a mum, are moments that can drive us into some challenging emotions, ones which were likely already there from our own baby, birth and childhood experiences, as well as lifetimes before then. But let's not get too caught up in that for now.

What motherhood and the journey towards it opens up is an opportunity to know your true self; to explore all the thoughts and emotions that rise up and to understand where they came from and why you think what you know about yourself. Why you are feeling the way you feel and discovering what lies beneath all the conditioning and life layers of who you should or should not be or what you should or should not do. 'Mums don't do that' is a common phrase that makes you question who you are. Yes, do question who you are. Explore yourself deeply because it's you who wishes to and not because someone else does. Just because it's always been that way, as far as anyone can remember, doesn't mean it's the right way. It's time for you to choose what is right for you.

Remembering who you are is really what we are all here on this planet for – to remember we are love. It is through the darkness of the womb, the darkness we can experience on our journey through the womb to yourself, and if it's your choice, to motherhood, that we ultimately come to the light. Once anyone – male or female – makes the decision to peel back the hurts, beliefs, and conditioning in the quest for awareness, they begin their journey to wholeness.

The mother wound, I believe, is not the mother sacrificing herself for her children. It is the children sacrificing themselves, their truth, their essence, for the mother, in order to stay safe. Children stifle who they are so as not to risk triggering the very person they need and love, no matter what style of mothering they experience. This means that you sacrificed yourself as the child, as did your mother and her mother before her and so on, from which there is unresolved healing. The more we as women can turn off the triggers, recognise and meet our own needs, be our own mothers and recognise our true selves, fulfil our own needs, and demand them, not only transforms your life, but the life of your children and future children. The more we can each release our own inner child from any dark and stifled place they may be in, the more all children will feel free – to be free. This is the same for men.

Imagine a world where children feel safe to be themselves. Imagine a world where you as a conscious parent are parenting from your self-aware adult self and not your hurt child self or your mum's hurt and frustrated child self. This is what the baby souls waiting to arrive, and those already here, are encouraging us to do. That their mum and dad can know them as the unique souls they are, free and safe to express all of who they are, without risk of censure for fear of triggering their parents to react from their own past hurts.

The truth is, we all have to take responsibility for our own sense of self, for how we feel. No one else is able to fill the holes of disempowerment or loss of self. No child is responsible for how their mother feels, or for trying to 'fix' her.

Take a moment to feel into where you may have been giving yourself a hard time, telling yourself you can't or you're rubbish or limiting yourself. Then ask yourself if you wish your child and future child to feel these limitations. To feel themselves as not good enough, or failures or wrong. Harsh, isn't it? You are your own worst critic and it's time to find new ways of knowing and loving yourself.

## The truth of you, the light, and birthing the light

As I continued to write this book and receive messages from Rosa, I finally understood why she described anyone drawn to this book as a 'Mother Mary'. You are birthing the light or are here to play a role in holding and growing this light. As a woman you are a portal between realms, able to receive love in its purest form and birth new consciousness, new life – how did we ever buy into the idea that we are of less value? We do the best we can with what we know, and then we grow. And then we rise – together.

Mother Mary is mentioned quite often throughout this book, her loving energy flowing through every word. But I feel it's important to ask you to question what you have been told about her. Who was put in charge of telling her story and what was their purpose? Remember, all is not as it seems and we are being asked to find our own truths.

In my mind, the biblical story of Mother Mary shows how this energy of women sacrificing themselves for the greater good has played out. Mother Mary is portrayed, mostly by male writers of a certain era, and most certainly from the 15th century, as virginal, pure, and self-sacrificing in order to bring in the light that was Christ. She sacrificed, she experienced loss, and is celebrated for her suffering amid it all. According to this version of the story, as women, this is who we should aspire to be and act. Certainly in the Western world.

So when we are not acting pure and virginal and self-sacrificing, or even feel like being those things, there is also a huge unconscious pressure that we're somehow wrong, we're not living up to this illusory ideal woman. You can see where the inner conflict lies; where the sacrifice lies. Because being like Mother Mary, as she has been portrayed not just as the Mother but the virgin mother in many texts, is not who we are, and I am daring to say, not who she was and is either. From my own moments with Mary and through other's channellings, I believe Mary was trained in the arts of sacred sex in the temples of Isis.

As women we are also wild and sexual and fierce in our love to live our best life, to create our best potential and create life, whatever way that is for you. And the pressure to be an image of someone, knowingly or unknowingly, a false impression set by someone else's beliefs and opinions, is the wound of the mother. Where you feel you are not allowed to be yourself. Where you sacrifice yourself in your desire to fit in with an impression of what you should be like. And all this coming from the control over the feminine that slowly, slowly took away the magnificence of creation and ability to create, and made it something to be ashamed of and something to suffer for.

These ancient beliefs are embedded deep in the psyche, and it is our responsibility as individuals to discover, re-discover, our own truths and not what we have been told to be true. In channelled meditations in the Divine Mother Meditation circle I run, both Christ and Mother Mary, among other representations of the Divine Mother energy, have brought healing to these ancient notions of sacrifice and suffering – this was not their truth but a truth that has been imposed on them. Both these energies said there was no sacrifice, they gave up nothing, they simply gave. Sacrifice and suffering have no place in the New Earth.

Their truth is unconditional love, not judgement or more than or less than, just love. When you can free yourself of the stories you hold, your own and those you've been told, and explore your emotions, the energy behind your beliefs and experiences, that is love, self-love, then the effect on you and the world is unimaginably beautiful.

## How does the word Mother make you feel?

I also feel it's important to ask you to feel into the word 'mother'. As with all words, it is loaded with whatever our thoughts, sub-conscious programmes and experiences are. Maybe you had a difficult relationship with your own mother, for example, and so this word may bring up negative thoughts and emotions. A challenging mother relationship is one of the most powerful blocks to becoming a mother yourself. Why would you want to be a mother when the very word and meaning has become distorted? The word may bring your body into stress and contraction.

Knowing that you most likely chose your parents and experiences on a soul level, as you'll read in this book, helps empower you to healing through the traumas and negative emotions of your childhood. Your challenges can become your greatest gifts and talents for you to rise into the natural, powerful mother energy you hold within, being wholly you as a mother, making choices from your whole self and not carrying the wounds of your own mother and likely hers before her, and so on. Imagine this truth of you?

For one of my clients, the distorted Mother energy came from a difficult Catholic school experience and a headteacher, the Mother Superior, who was bullying and often told my client how useless she was. She understandably drew back from the word mother and had an upside-down view of what it meant to be a mother. She didn't want to be associated with this wounded mother energy.

So if it's helpful, write down the word mother on a piece of paper, notice how you feel and begin writing all the adjectives that come to mind, positive and negative on what this means to you.

The Divine Mother energy that flows through this book is simply pure, unconditional love. The only way I can describe this energy is wholeness. In this energy, you feel safe, held and loved without question or judgement, no matter what you perceive you have done that's good or bad. The image I have of this energy is a woman standing tall, watching the world and its people and all we get up to through the gaze of love. Not telling them what's right or wrong but being there as a guide and loving space as and when each of us is ready to grow through our perceived mistakes, harm and hurts. She is here to support you in your self-awareness, to become the best version of you that you wish for. She provides a safe, loving space to help you become who you already are: love.

Take a moment to feel into this energy. You are it, you hold it, it's in everything and everyone, everywhere, it's just that the layers of lifetimes have buried it deep. Have no doubt, however, that it's there. And your journey through this book will support you in feeling this more and more. As you read these words I'm asking for the Divine Mothers to hold you in unconditional love, feel this.

## The layers of you, the layers of this book and your relationship with them

The messages and spiritual insights in this book build in layers, starting with our individual healing and eventually revealing what this actually means for the collective, the world and yes, even the Universe – you are that powerful!

This book also brings the spiritual and practical together by examining thought patterns and beliefs that not only affect you personally but also affect your journey to motherhood. It covers how you can transform your conditioning to bring about changes in yourself and to your experiences, and how to transform them. It offers ways of connecting with your higher self and your babies.

Connection to all things, channelling, feeling, knowing, seeing energy is not just for the few, it's for all of us, we've just been trained out of this norm. Our natural state of being is to be connected, follow our intuition and gut instinct, our hearts, rather than be caught up in the programming and logic of our minds. We've just been trained otherwise, told that the mind and logic is all. Of course, there's a place for logic, but I would argue: where has this got us if that's all we're operating from? We're missing out on the fullness of who we are if we only try and figure things out using our logical brain.

Old form spirituality hasn't helped with this feeling of separation by often taking on the old pattern of the Church, where only an ordained person had the power and authority to 'speak with God' or share 'the words of the Almighty' and dictate the rules. Old school spirituality followed this pattern in that there were a few 'special ones' who then shared the information, as if only special people had the skill and right to do this. I hope through this book you will begin to feel your own specialness and magic. Know that you are special, you have the right to connect, an innate gift to do so, if you choose. There will be a couple of exercises throughout this book and listed at the end that will help you with this. You are extraordinary in your ordinariness.

The one thing above all else that I would wish you to take away from this book is to know at your very core that you are not stuck, you are not your thoughts or experiences, and you are not alone. You are never alone. You are loved beyond measure and there is always, always a bigger picture. Hold onto this truth amid turbulent times. You are already the love that you seek.

This book explores the journey to motherhood and the core healing that lies within it for each of us, the collective, our future babies, and Mother Earth.

# The individual

The journey to motherhood can often be the catalyst to awaken to a bigger picture – the notion that we are more than a body with physical and material needs. The trauma, the grief, anger, frustration, the why me – the 'what have I done to deserve this'– type questions, can keep us focused on the negative.  Be open to see how new learning can lead you down the path of inner exploration.

This book is here to support you on your journey. It will guide you to look within to find the answers to your questions and offers a very different perspective – the perspective of the baby spirit world and of your babies themselves.

Just as we have our own unique path in life and choice in how we live it, so too do our babies. The spirit I call Rosa offers us this insight and healing through her words in this book.

I am yet to fully discover, or  more likely allow myself to discover, who Rosa is and her role in my life and yours. I hope that by the end of this book we may have discovered this together. For I am merely writing the words that come through me rather than waiting to be 'ready', rather than waiting for the right time, the right knowledge, the right information. I trust that all is happening exactly as it should.

In my eyes, Rosa is my baby soul, whom I released on 5 December 2010, in a heart-breaking, life-changing moment of choice. I had no idea at the time, in my sense of 'evilness', unworthiness, victimhood, and grief, that she was so much more than that. That I was so much more than that.

Our story, I hope, will open your hearts and minds to the full glory of this life on earth and what it means for each and every one of us, on an individual, collective, and spiritual level.

# Chapter 1
# Soul Awakening Journey to Motherhood

No matter what your background, no matter what you think is possible or impossible for you, know that there are no limits to your dreams and your heart's desires. If we could realise in one instant all of who we are or what we are here on this earth for, I seriously think our minds would be blown.

From the moment of conception, if not before, in fact definitely before, each and every step we take, whether we think it's random, whether we judge it a good step or a bad one, is leading us to exactly where we need to be. As we frequently say in spiritual groups, it is not the destination, it's the journey. However irritating that can sound, it is the moment-by-moment decisions we make that create the outcomes we have to live with that are important.

If you feel called to it, please take some time to write down your journey so far and ask what the lessons have been. Or review a past experience to look again at the lesson you may have missed at the time. If we lose the lesson, it may keep coming back until we recognise it. Notice which thoughts and emotions keep coming back, with a sense of curiosity. Where have those experiences taken you? Who do you blame? Who are you angry at? Or are you blaming yourself? Are you playing the martyr or the victim? When was the very first time you felt them? We all have these stories playing out in our minds and they are so very far from the truth of you, the light of you. And those stories can change as you recognise and accept the hugely powerful soul that you are.

Be curious and honest with yourself about your journey to motherhood – what is it bringing you? What is it teaching you about yourself? What emotions is it bringing up? What are you telling yourself about yourself – and are these beliefs yours or someone else's? How well are they serving you?

As the amazing Louise Hay said, "In order to clean the house, you first need to see the dirt." There is no more running from ourselves;

it is time to face ourselves, see the dirt, and wipe it away so you can see, truly see, how much you shine. How does that sound?

Our journey to motherhood can often be the catalyst for our spiritual awakening, as it was for me.

## Who am I to write this book?

I work now as a spiritual guide, healer, spirit baby medium, and intuitive soul purpose channel, working between the worlds helping women to find themselves and meet their babies – helping women to know themselves as miracles equal to those of their babies. I am honoured to be able to 'see', 'hear', and sense energy; to read energy with anyone's permission. I am able to travel to whichever realm or time your soul energy wishes to take you to and discover any root wounds, past, ancestral, life between life experiences that may be pushing on you now that you are ready to see and find resolution to in order for you to own more of you and step forward more powerfully as, you.

I urge you to see yourself as magical, miracle creators; portals of life. But I am a 'normal' girl who has lived a 'normal' life. I grew up on the rough end of a housing estate, thankfully on the beautiful island of Jersey, with two inspiring, gifted and, of course, often annoying brothers.

My dad was fun, loving, and supportive. He broke new ground as being a very hands-on dad and husband for that time in the 70s, when men were men and didn't change nappies. He was a youth worker with his own family history of demons that eventually took hold of him in the form of alcohol. It took time but eventually I gained a clear understanding which led to forgiveness of the high soul he is. I believe a soul whose purpose was to change his ancestral pattern, and therefore my family line, of the strict patriarchal rules and beliefs of English northern men from a mining background where a beating with a belt was viewed as good parenting. By being a loving, hands-on dad, he did his absolute best to go against the grain of his own ancestors, upbringing, and experience, and did his utmost to free us and our own children from the 'sins of the fathers'. It's a huge task to try and break the mould of patriarchy where women are seen as 'less than' and children treated as if they didn't have feelings or dreams of their own. Being brought up with strong, loving female mentors in the form of his aunts, I believe, helped him in his task. In my experience it's never too late to make sense of how we were raised, and to extract and interpret the gifts and learning from how we were parented. To try and understand what our parents are teaching us, especially if they do not fit the ideal.

And my mum was and is the strongest, most fiercely loving, wise, giving, and fair-minded woman I have ever been blessed to meet. I chose well. Looking back now, her determination to not inflict the mother wound on us left us with a lot of freedom but also often lostness as to what life was all about and what we were about. Rarely were we told what to do or think, apart from the obvious safety guidance. Mostly her response to questions was: do what you feel is right – not think is right.

I didn't always get it then. I wanted someone to tell me what to do; that would have been so much easier. It also left me with the belief, or rather I took on the belief, that I had to do it all by myself. However, when my brothers and I inevitably made the 'wrong' choices, my mum was always there to pick us back up again. Being a mum now I can see how extremely difficult this path of keeping out of the way and letting us children find our own way must have been for her. She was determined not to inflict her own stuff onto us. I asked her about her parenting style when she was over in London visiting us, only a week before her very unexpected and shocking passing. It was almost like we both knew, without knowing, that we wouldn't get to chat this deeply again. "I loved it all. I love you all." There were difficult moments and many worrying moments, but not once did she feel she had lost out. "I didn't own you," she said. "I had no right to interfere with your choices or stifle you. You're here to make your own life." She didn't sacrifice, she said, she gave. I am doing my best but still working up to this way of mothering – with perhaps a little more balance in the guidance area! A growth and breakthrough of generational patterns of parenting through my own family.

I wasn't one of those kids who have always seen angels and fairies or dead people, not that I remember, at least. But I always had a sense of something 'other'. When I was about seven, I remember having a conversation with my parents that God couldn't possibly be this old bloke in the sky with a beard and a switchboard answering all our calls for help and choosing which ones he had time or care for. For one, why would 'he', God, have to choose who to help?

I concluded to my parents there and then that it was all energy. And when we prayed or asked for help we were sending out good thoughts and positive energy, to that person.

And I distinctly remember saying: I want to heal the world! A rather grand statement for a seven-year-old, but this is what I came out with when asked what I wanted to do in life.

At that time I had no idea what that meant or entailed. I just wanted people to be kind to each other and be happy. I was convinced this was possible somehow.

Wherever this grand ideal came from, it gradually became something I forgot about or, at the very least, kept to myself. It's not like I was an angelic child who never upset anyone and was always kind – far from it. It's one aspect I've had to face – the part that was mean – and be able to forgive myself for.  If we seek change, we can use everyday events that challenge us to find out what lies beneath. We're all learning as we go.

However, it's only recently I've connected this memory of wanting to change the world, heal the world, to how it must have always been in the background guiding my choices. Perhaps it was this that led me to travel to many places in the world and meet people from all sorts of cultures and backgrounds to try and understand the world and its people more. These adventures eventually led to a degree in Anthropology and Development Studies and a career in journalism so I could share all that was going on in this wonderful, but often seemingly harsh, world.

My fascination with the workings of the world led me to a Masters in Violence, Conflict and Development, after which, I joined an international charity. As a media officer, I could focus solely on trying to communicate not only the injustices that go on but also the stories of inspirational people across the globe who, either in spite of their own intense suffering or because of it, really are making a difference and making the world a better place for others.

I hadn't joined up my thinking at this stage or contemplated looking at the bigger picture. I never once related any of this to personal healing or healing of an individual and definitely not to spiritual healing or part of a greater plan. It was an intellectual pursuit and a career that was very fulfilling but I took nothing more from it.

I'd always been intrigued by the non-tangible though – palm reading was one of my party tricks from the age of eighteen, and even I used to be a bit taken aback by the accuracy of some of the readings.

It's funny looking back now and remembering all this because none of it really registered at the time. I had plenty of signs over the years that there was something 'more' going on than the world we could see, some of them quite dramatic and literally life-saving messages.

I'd always wanted to travel and looking back I wonder what I was running away from – or to. What I was trying to find. I ended up in Egypt three times and even considered studying Egyptology I was so fascinated by the culture. I felt at home on the streets of Cairo and in the pyramids and temples. Now I know I'm connected to Isis and Mother Mary it makes far more sense in hindsight. It doesn't matter what the reason for my travel bug was, I guess, because I obviously found what I was looking for: all aspects of life, the good, the bad, the beautiful, and the ugly. The adventure, the loneliness, the fear, the threat of living and dying, and the utter beauty of the world and its people.

I did ponder why people live such different lives – why some were rich and some were poor, some were happy, some mean – but I did no more than ponder. I know I had a number of angelic experiences when travelling, the most profound one being when I was in Morocco camping in the wilderness. My first ever overseas trip when I was eighteen.

As my three girlfriends and I were deciding where to set up camp, I heard a very strong NO! I was rooted to the spot. I physically couldn't move. I told my friends we needed to find a hotel – we would find the money or plead to be let in – but going down to camp among the trees alone was really not a good idea.

They listened, but our minds and lack of money at that time led us to camp in that beautiful spot. As the four of us prepared food and ate and shacked up in a tiny tent by the river, surrounded by trees, all seemed well and I dismissed my message as me just being a scaredy-cat.

Until, in the later hours of the evening as darkness fell, along came Diable. Diable – meaning devil in French – came in the form of a desperate guy trying to make the most of life before Ramadan. He wanted drugs – hashish. We had a tiny bit but for some reason chose not share it. We just wanted him to go and our eighteen-year-old good-girl selves didn't want to admit to anyone else we were trying out one of the local delicacies.

Years later, as part of my job working for an international charity and travelling to often desperate places, I underwent training on being kidnapped. The first lesson I learned if threatened: always give them what they want. They can take anything and it won't matter, but your life cannot be replaced. But at eighteen, and fresh from a small island with zero street sense, neither I nor my friends knew this.

When we refused, he proclaimed himself to be Diable and he would burn us down inside our tent with the candle we had lit outside it. I was quite fearless at the time and jumped out shouting – we all shouted – but of course, there was not a person, a house, village or town in sight. We were alone.

All our shouting in the world wasn't going to raise the alarm or chase him away. In fact, it only made him angrier and he grabbed me and held a long, curved knife to my throat. Eventually, he released me and I returned to the tent to tell the girls. We knew, unless we absolutely had to fight for our lives, there was no point resisting right now. We simply surrendered to the situation.

We began writing letters of apology to our mums and dads for being so stupid and getting ourselves killed! And then the strangest most miraculous thing happened. In our surrender there came a sense of peace. I felt protected and safe and knew we would come to no harm. I could see Diable for what he was – a scared and desperate man – not an evil man.

Such was our sense of peace, two of my friends even fell asleep. Whilst I and my friend Julie stayed awake. As she plaited my hair into lots of tiny braids to pass the time, we talked to this guy as best we could. We made a connection, made ourselves human, made him human and the fear vanished.

Without the fear, what was his story? What was our story? We shared bread and cheese (but still didn't share the hashish!) and stayed up all night. He left as the sun rose – and so did we. Packed up the tent in record time and got out of there and onto the first bus that stopped on the nearest road. There is much more to this story, but what is relevant is the sense of absolutely knowing that we were safe, we were protected, and that even if we died, that was okay too.

Acceptance of our situation dramatically changed the energies around it. And that was the very first lesson in which I became aware of the power of working with energy, the angelic realms and the importance of connection. Not that I realised any of this at the time. It was just a great story and we'd survived and went on to enjoy another month of adventure in this beautiful country with its beautiful people.

I think we all did eventually tell our parents many, many years later. But that is the spirit of youth – the taking of risks and dealing with the consequences to manage them better next time. To be free, to live life to the fullest. So why as adults do we seem to lose this spirit of adventure? Why does the fear kick in and we become small, start playing it small, and fitting in?

## What's your healer's journey?

Everything we do is relevant to remembering who we are, what we are here to uncover and learn about ourselves, and how we choose to show up in the world. Perhaps take a moment to write down what's brought you to where you are and what's brought you to this book.

It took me until my forties to see that my journalist and media officer careers were the most perfect training ground for being a messenger – because I've actually always been a messenger. Asking questions and reporting back various different messages and opinions and stories from the inauthentic politician to truly inspiring Rwandan genocide survivors.

Not once did I question printing their messages – this was my job, my role – and it was not my role to put my words in their mouth or censor them in any way. And so here I am, still a messenger, a journalist if you like, for the higher realms.

At the time, however, I didn't really look deeply into these angelic encounters and messages. I was intrigued but didn't question them, nor was I actually surprised – I simply shrugged them off, grateful that I'd had an insight that had helped in a particular situation. I hadn't the awareness of, or the readiness to look into, such experiences as part of a bigger, more profound picture. We all come to that in our time and for our own reasons.

It took the deeply upsetting loss of Rosa to make me really look at life, the why and the how; essentially, the meaning of life, why things happen and why we're here.

It wasn't too many months after Rosa's funeral that my intention to understand why caused things to happen. My best friend Sam gave me Lorna Byrne's book Angels in My Hair, as it has a chapter about miscarriage. My counsellor at the time also said I was approaching the loss of Rosa from a very spiritual perspective – and another light went on. She suggested I read the book Many Lives, Many Masters by Brian Weiz.

Well, that was it – I was off on my journey. I was introduced to the concept of synchronicities, and what seemed to be chance meetings eventually led me to the Balham Spiritualist Church. There I saw my first medium in action. This was followed by the College of Psychic Studies and finally to the Holistic Healing College.

The moment I knew, really knew, at the core of my being that there was a 'God', a Source, a something much bigger and other than me, was when I was sitting on the 355 bus from Tooting to Balham in London, heading to the Spiritualist Church, and musing about what I might hear or learn. In that unexpected moment, my life and my world opened up in a profound way. There are no words really to describe what happened on that 355 bus – but to say – I just knew. I simply knew I wasn't alone. There was a greater force, a loving one, and everything was going to be okay.

I studied spiritual counselling at the Holistic Healing College, thinking if I learnt these techniques I could help others who had been through similar pregnancy and loss situations. If I learnt these techniques I could help others' heal their wounds.

For the first four modules, I actively took notes, soaked up the reading, and asked myself how a particular module might help someone. I got frustrated with Qigong because I couldn't see how I was going to be able to learn this and do this practice with someone to help them. True to form, I was pursuing it from an intellectual, analytical point of view. It was only at the fifth module when I asked a fellow student where they saw themselves going after the course, and their reply was, "I'm still going through my own healing to think about that." The penny suddenly dropped, it's vital to heal yourself first.

I'd been too busy watching the world as an observer rather than a participant, and in this case too busy going through the modules, rather than engaging in any personal healing processes. I'm guessing my stance of, "I'm fine, I don't need healing", which I genuinely believed at that time, was actually a way of avoiding the uncomfortable feelings. But once I'd opened myself up to the possibility of growth, the shift was remarkable.

Childhood experiences may cut us off from our emotions, but it is our emotions that are our signposts to what is true, what is right for us, and what is very wrong for us. Signposts which highlight all those aspects of ourselves crying out to be noticed.

And so here I am now, having written this book. We have to allow our journeys to unfold step by step because our minds can only take us so far with what we think is possible. Part of a message that came through for a gifted client, Michael, a super cool musician, very much of the new Divine Masculine breed of man, that he is happy for me to share is:

*"Your mind will only tell you where you have been and not where you are headed."*

# Chapter 2
## Rosa's Story, Rosa's Choice

It has taken ten years from the moment I made my decision to release Rosa to writing this book. The inspiration for the book, however, came to me in 2016. I was sitting having a drink with two of my gorgeous work colleagues at this time. I had confessed the whole story to one of them; the other knew the surface story. For some reason, perhaps because we had opened a second bottle of wine, when she asked me what had happened, I felt able to tell her. When she asked me how I felt about it now, I replied, "I am so grateful it happened. It's changed my life. Rosa changed my life."

Saying those words lit something up in me. How on earth could I now be feeling grateful for an experience that had almost destroyed me? This is amazing, I thought, and slightly bonkers. Have I totally lost it? How have I come from a place of depression, anger, sadness, feeling like a failure and a 'bad' person, useless, not good enough, not deserving, in need of being punished and full of shame, the list goes on, to the point I never felt able to tell the 'truth' of what had happened, to being not only very happy in life but grateful for it all?

On the tube home, I wrote these words on a scrap of paper: "Never in a million years would I have thought I would be grateful for choosing to release my baby." And suddenly there it was: the knowing that it was Rosa's choice too; the book, the title, the cover and the purpose – healing for all women on their journeys to motherhood – all there in my mind's eye. My first conscious, albeit slightly tipsy, experience of channelling Rosa.

Even with this new purpose, I had not stepped into my power or my gifts at this time. I put it out there to the universe to connect me with a medium or a channel who would write Rosa's side of the story. Never did I imagine that I would be doing this myself. Every medium I saw said they could only reach Rosa through their guides because she was such a high soul, and couldn't connect with her directly.

By then, I knew I was bringing through messages for people during the Soul Plan Readings I was doing. I also knew I was connecting with what I refer to as Source energy or Creator energy, or the energy of All that is. And the image of this book kept floating into my mind until one day I thought – why not see if I can talk to Rosa!

And so I did.

Here are my first tentative questions and Rosa's very first words with me. Her side of the story complements my own, which you have read above.

> **Rosa**: You need to write my words as I express them and don't question them no matter how much your ego is screaming out for me to stop.

> **Me**: When?

> **Rosa**: I am ready now – are you? We are going to heal the world with this book, you and I, as we are going to bring through some spiritual truths that have yet to be heard. Be prepared, for some may not be ready, but it is time and you won't be alone. There are many who are ready and therefore open to a whole new pathway to being in this world.

> **Me**: Are you sure?

> **Rosa**: You don't have to take this on in this lifetime. It is a choice you made and one that no one is holding you to.

> **Me**: Is this safe for my family?

> **Rosa**: We are your family and they will have no clue what you are doing until it is done and then they will be ready and they will be proud.

> **Me**: How?

> **Rosa**: We can play – we need to play as this is big stuff happening here and it's important to get it right so people hear the truth of the message. Maybe we do start with me as I can begin the story and lead you into a comfortable place

where you can start from your human view. Let's do that.

I came to this earth to seek love, but all I found was selfishness and greed. It was not a world I liked the look of and so I chose a vessel that was not whole, the likelihood being I would be released when I was ready to return to my true mission of uplifting the world and baring my soul to the masses through this kind soul who offered me her heart and her mind.

Her body was not ready for me and so it is that together we began to raise our vibration so we would one day connect in the realm of spirit and she would channel my words and my life to lift you all with the truths of the cosmos.

It is not through her body that she served me, but in a far more powerful and meaningful way, by lifting her vibration to meet me where I am, and so in turn lift the world.

Do not be afraid, little one. This may not have been what you were expecting, but it is what is happening. Take a deep breath and go with me with love; the love you showed me all those many years ago when you accepted my spirit and then let me go.

For that was the greatest gift you gave me, as you knew in your heart I was not meant for this world. You heard me and you answered me. There were many other things you could be doing with your life rather than bringing up a high spirit in the body of a child who is damaged and not able to express its frustrations and limited in the truths it could tell.

I was never meant to be in that world and I knew you would never allow that to happen, because you love me beyond measure and therefore let me go.

I have already lived lifetimes locked in chains and I have learnt that lesson many times until I became perfect at it. I do not need to learn this lesson anymore. You, however, are on a lesson to learn about love, love in all its forms, and letting go of love is indeed one of those lessons that can tear you apart.

I know this was difficult for you and a little bit torn apart you became. However, you did not fully crumble, because you knew I was with you. I was with you on the tube that day – and see how that lightened your day. I am not a figment of your imagination. I am real, I am here, I am Rosa, and this is my story told through the gift of love that we have for each other.

I am your guide and your mentor and we have never been apart. It is not often our guides come to earth with us, but you were being so stubborn and shut down all of your beliefs and intuition about me and God, that I took that drastic action of risking all for you.

I knew you would not keep me chained, but I also didn't know that, because circumstances are not always right and something or someone may have convinced you otherwise. However, all that was put in your path were souls who cared and comforted you and also knew the bigger story that was going on here, so no one would have persuaded you otherwise.

Yes, at times you have been easily led by the will of others and the shame they induced in you as your weak spots were triggered into pleasing people who do not deserve to be pleased by you, for they are only showing you where you need to take back your power.

I didn't fully understand Rosa's words at the time, but I do now. She was letting me know that by not staying – or as she described at one point: being trapped in the physical world – meant I was encouraged – kicked rather brutally, I would say – into my own healing journey. One that would enable me to shed all those layers of shame and grief, anger and resentment, and literally lighten up and raise my vibration so I could do what I'm doing now.

There was much more for Rosa to say at this point, but my husband, Lee, walked in and he must have thought I was doing something dodgy as I looked so shell-shocked. When I tried to explain what was happening, he was the one who was shell-shocked.

He has been and always will be my greatest, most loving cheerleader. But he will admit that there were many times he was a little worried about my mental state and had to double-check I was still the woman he had married.

He may not be fully with me on the soul-exploring front as yet, but he is more comfortable now with me zipping about the universe and talking with beings he can't see. I know it is a look of awe and not weirdness I see in his eyes when I share the photos of the babies now arrived in the world; the babies I'd already met in spirit when they were just a mum's knowing wish and not yet a physical reality.

He is more open to the possibility that we have access to all the information we need and are meant to know – we are not on this journey alone and neither were we ever meant to be. It is simply the times and culture that have allowed for this disconnect to seem normal, when in fact it is the connection and how it was eons ago that is rising again to bring about a new way for the planet. One of unity and connection.

It wasn't, however, only my husband who was questioning what was happening. I was questioning myself – a lot. I didn't feel desperate or mad or even sad any longer about my own journey to motherhood. In Rosa's message, she mentioned that I had seen her on the tube that day. I live in London and when I went back to work six weeks after releasing her, I was zoning out as you do and suddenly I had the clearest, most beautiful image of her in my mind's eye. She showed herself to me as a girl of about four or five years old, with brown hair in a bob style, deep brown smiling eyes, and the biggest grin. I'd like to say I noticed the colour of her clothes, but I didn't take that in. It all happened in an instant and then she was gone. It was more the feeling I had in that moment that took my breath away.

Firstly, I just knew it was Rosa, which is pretty hard to understand. Secondly, I knew that she was happy, she was fine and she was with me. It was a feeling, an instant healing if you like, as I was re-entering the real world after my six-week bubble and absence from work and the anxiety that can bring up. I felt a sense of peace and knew I was okay, that everything was going to be okay.

It was a feeling and image that I held in my mind and heart; that immediate and intimate sense of connection and knowing I tried hard to re-create in the weeks ahead. But it was a long time – over a year – before I managed to feel her energy again. I have not 'seen' Rosa again, only felt her very powerful presence. As I developed my channelling, my seeing became a hearing of her words.

As I delved deeper into myself, clearing out more and more of my own 'baggage' I hadn't even known I was carrying, I experienced greater peace and acceptance of my journey. I was excited about my gifts and the potential this provided for helping other women. The old me held the thought that I was some grieving madwoman making all of this up. I had to learn to trust myself and my intuition, to trust Rosa and the Universe, which was a huge learning curve. I would say it's taken me three years to get to where I am now; to open up to trusting the messages from Rosa for this book and those for the women and men who I'm working with and supporting on their own journeys to parenthood.

On this journey of discovery, and dipping in and out of doubt about what is or isn't real, I am blessed to be surrounded by hugely loving, like-minded and magical people, whose presence lifts and heals myself and others. Their insights confirming my own.

## Can you communicate with your baby and loved ones in spirit, the trees, your pets?

I'm often asked now to teach people how to channel or teach them to become spirit baby communicators but I haven't felt the call just yet. I realised it's not something you can teach, there's no logical method: if you do A you'll get to B. Yes there are many exercises and practices that will strengthen your psychic and intuitive senses but I believe the key to opening up your gifts is removing all the blocks and beliefs that lead you to believe you can't or it's not possible. We're all unique and the way I do it is not necessarily right for anyone else. I was never trained, it wasn't a gift I ever imagined I had, it just happened one day. And it wasn't' whilst sitting in silence after meditating for hours in a kaftan and practising it.

My less-than-glamorous first moment of being aware of channelling energy was when I stopped off at a pub on the way home from work for some peace and quiet so I could write up a soul plan I'd promised to do as a freebie for one of my neighbours. I wasn't yet charging for my readings as I was still practising – or rather, not feeling confident enough to charge at the time. This pub had a scrubby old garden. I knew no one sat in there so I could grab a coffee and it would be quiet, some me time.

As I sat there looking at my friend's soul plan chart and starting to write down what I could remember about the various energies, it was like I wasn't in charge of the pen after a while. All these words and language that I would never use were flowing out onto the page. I could hear the words in my mind, whilst also hear my own thoughts asking what on earth was happening. It was a bit disconcerting but I kept going with it and streams and streams of information were flowing through me. It was dark and I was freezing by this time but I didn't want to break the spell.

It felt like I was under a spell, sat in the pub garden freezing, but also not sat in the pub garden, the whole energy around me was like nothing I'd ever experienced. Now I know that I was feeling the energy of my Soul Plan guides surrounding me and they were working through me. So, had I done anything differently that day to any other day? No. It was just my time. And if you choose to have a time like this, it will happen.

Each and every person can connect and channel information and guidance from the many light beings around them and your higher self. Your higher self is the part of your soul that vibrates on a higher level. It is the eternal and unlimited part of you that knows everything about you and holds all the information you need to know, guides your ideas, inspirations and choices, and excites you. Your higher self only talks in simple love language, unlike the ego part of yourself which is a heavier energy and can be highly critical and complicated.

You are already channelling, you channel every day. Those moments of inspiration when you're in the shower, for example, when an idea pops into your head, or you suddenly know the solution to a problem. Artists, musicians, writers, whenever you are creating, this is you channelling energy. Your mind is rarely involved. Einstein was a great one for saying intuition, not logic, was the way to create solutions. Start to notice the difference between your ego-mind decisions and your higher-mind or heart decisions. This will strengthen your intuition and creative communication channels.

My one suggestion when moving from your everyday channelling to intentionally connecting with other beings is to always set the intention of connecting in with only those beings of the purest, unconditionally loving light, for your highest and best good.

So instead of training someone to be a channel or spirit baby communicator, what I prefer to do is guide someone to having more belief and confidence in themselves that they are worthy and absolutely able to connect with any energy they wish. Help them find out what beliefs, blocks, fears and traumas they have around being open to discovering their hidden gifts or able to communicate in this way. Thoughts such as: is it possible? Is it weird? Will I be judged for it? What if I can't do it? What if I can do it? Or, I'm terrified of it. Past life experiences can really play out here in feeling safe to connect and step into your power and your gifts because at one point in time you may well have been punished for it. Think witches for example. They weren't witches, they were powerful women. As each block comes to light, why they're there and where they've come from, the clearer you become on your fears and traumas, heal and move through them – the clearer your connection.

Freewriting is such a powerful way of getting out of your own head and allowing words to stream through you. They don't even need to make sense, go with the experience of freely writing and notice how you feel.

You may be long into your connection journey or just starting out. If you're new to this, you may want to try this exercise now before we move onto the chapters on conception and baby loss, so you feel you are not only a reader of someone else's words but empowered to free your own words and deep soul insight into how you feel when you're reading them and why. We can often feel so helpless on this journey to motherhood, that any tool you can draw on to bring yourself back to a place of more knowing and connection is hugely transformational. You are at the mercy of nothing and no one – you can take charge of how you feel about whatever you are experiencing. What is true for you or not. This is your power, no matter how deeply buried that may feel at times.

So, if you wish to, give yourself permission to take 20 minutes or so just for you. Create a space, just for you. That might include lighting a candle and creating an altar or it might not – wherever you are, YOU are. Wherever you are, your babies are.

Take three deep breaths, imagining you're breathing in the light and this light is moving all the way around your head, down your spine to your feet, and back up to breathe out.

On the third breath let out a deep sigh and allow the weight of your mind to slip down into your chest, your heart chakra.

From your heart, command your energy to zero point. Then command your energy to ground, and finally command your energy to Source.

Set the intention of connecting in with pure unconditional love of Source and imagine yourself sitting under a waterfall of light, cleaning and cleansing your energy and surrounding you in love.

You can ask to connect in with your spirit baby or your higher self or any light being for guidance on any question you may have, or just allow whatever it is that wants to flow through you to flow down the crown of your head, your arm, your hand and onto the page. Start writing, even if it feels like gobbledygook at first, it's a practice.

See how you go, like any muscle, you are strengthening your connection.

If you haven't done so already, it's also beautiful to write a letter to your baby in spirit, pouring out your heart to them. You can then burn this letter and allow the energy to drift up into the realms, either for releasing or with the intention of it reaching your spirit baby.

Something else you can play with when you feel low or confused is to light a candle and stare into the flame. Allow the light to help fizzle away any negative emotions. You can also ask to be shown visions in the flame too. And if you don't have a candle, your imagination is everything. Close your eyes and imagine gazing into the flame, it's the same effect.

I hope these two exercises will help support you on your journey through this book and beyond. I'll share another spirit baby practice with you further on and you can access my guided meditations, the links to which are at the back of the book.

# Chapter 3
# Baby Loss
# Why do babies choose not to stay?
# Discover their 'why'

As the months went by, I continued to practise my channelling and connecting in with Rosa – the messages you will read throughout this book. The more I set the intention of connecting with her, the easier it became. It didn't matter where I was, at home, in the park or in a café, I'd started learning how to tune everything else out and to 'hear' and 'see' her words and messages.

Being in a coffee shop is a great practice actually for your connection as you tune your ears to hearing only what you want to hear. Like you're leaning in to hear a friend's voice over clattering cups and background noise. It helps you focus.

By now, I was helping other women to heal their experiences of baby loss, by guiding them through their trauma and releasing any of those more destructive emotions such as guilt and helplessness. Because there is another truth to your experience and that is the truth held by your babies in spirit.

More and more often I was connecting in with the energy of spirit babies – those who had chosen not to stay and those who are yet to arrive. Again it was a practise in trusting what I was seeing and hearing, so if you wish to communicate with your babies, keep practising. Eventually your ego-mind will ease with questioning whether it's real or not.

Rosa is the high soul that allows this to happen – the middle woman if you like – inviting the baby spirits in to connect with me.

The bigger picture of why babies choose not to stay was becoming clearer. When I was going through my miscarriages, I barely spoke about them at the time. I felt I couldn't somehow. Not only did I not want to face how I felt, I also felt there was a stigma. No one seemed to understand, or didn't want to talk about it, because it made them feel uncomfortable – it made me feel uncomfortable.

Every time there was another baby announcement I felt a second of joy for them and then all this anger and envy rose up, why them and not me? I asked myself. This only served to make me kick myself even harder, because now I was convincing myself even more of what a horrible person I was because I couldn't be happy for someone else. Incidentally, when I was pregnant with Samuel, I felt the other side of this when someone at work who I was quite friendly with stopped talking to me. She knew nothing of my journey and her own experience of miscarriage led her to those same feelings of bitterness and her being unable to be near me and my growing bump. I believe now that being as open as we can about our experiences helps to lift the shame and the loss for others.

What we as women tell ourselves and how we treat ourselves after a miscarriage or a termination is all very different, and this is because we are filtering the event through our own unique life experiences.

For me, staying quiet and getting on with it, 'it's just one of those things', even after the third miscarriage, came from a place of always needing to be seen as strong, not allowing myself to be vulnerable and certainly not letting anyone else see me as vulnerable. I didn't need help. I could manage this on my own. People won't like me if they see I'm vulnerable, or I'll disappoint them, was one underlying belief and therefore it wasn't safe to be vulnerable.

Essentially, I didn't want to be seen, even by myself, because of the sense of unworthiness, feeling like a failure and that I didn't deserve to be a mum. I closed down, although I didn't recognise this at the time. I simply thought I was strong and getting on with it. There was no time to be weak.

This, of course, was far from the truth. I was merely repeating patterns, programmes and beliefs buried deep in my subconscious mind from childhood and before. All this I now know can be transformed, lifted off if you like, for each of us to discover who we really are.

My deepest wish is for every single woman who has lived through a miscarriage, termination or baby loss, to know that they don't have to feel the way they do. The experience does not define them or dictate their life because of the potential of acceptance and understanding. It may be hard to grasp right now, but at some point, when you are ready, when the time is right, you will find peace with your experience and yourself. And through grace, it will enhance your life as there is always a bigger picture and your babies very much have a choice in this.

My bigger picture is that after my fifth experience of baby loss, and subsequent healing journey, I discovered my life purpose – to support women to reconnect with themselves, their babies and future babies in spirit. I learned that it is possible to heal, that there is always, always a reason and that we are not on this journey to motherhood alone, but in it together with our babies.

My wish is for you to be able to understand your experience on a deeper level, understand yourself, understand your baby's journey, and to know that it was nothing you did or didn't do. It is not your fault and all really will be okay. Your babies are fine and in many cases come back when the time is right. And while we all of course wish for our babies to be with us, know that on some level they always are and are holding us in so much love.

For that is the truth.

I hope that the following words from Rosa about baby loss and her experience as she was released from this physical world will provide some comfort for you.


**Rosa's shares her experience of release**

I was so filled with joy as I could once again be whole. For part of me had stayed within you in order to keep this body of ours going and this was to ensure that it had to be your choice to release me. Yet at heart, it was the choice of us both for this to happen.

You did not know this at the time, and so you grieved and you shouted and you swore and you hated life. It has to be said that all of this had to happen in order for you to embrace life, my dear, for you were not embracing life at this time. You were living only some kind of half-life and it was to the fullness of life that you had to awaken.

I would wish to say sorry to you for this, but this too would be an untruth, for how can we be sorry for what has transpired from that moment? Don't you feel more alive than ever before, because of the death you have experienced? And yet I did not experience that death. I only experienced a short time of joy in the womb of your body and the love that I felt there. And it was at this time that it was tempting to stay, for it is good to be close to one another physically.

However, I also knew that this joy was to be short-lived, and the longer I stayed with you the harder it would be to leave. So we came to this choice together – that I must leave at that exact time, and yet it had to be you who was to make the choosing. For however much easier it would have been for me to up and go, and for you to be left dealing with the life that ended, this lesson of the world being against you, and the world being in control, was not one which we were learning. It was to the self that you had to make a choice.

To choose for yourself and by yourself the fate of yourself and your family and the other, that was me. To see that you do indeed have a choice and a say in how your world works and that each choice has a consequence and a reaction to that choice. To see that everything is not as it seems.

That it was not your husband's choice, or your son's choice, or the world's choice. It was indeed your choice. For you would not have coped with me as a physical being, knowing that the physical being was not one of action and perfection.

So you made your choice, as is your will and your right, and so I too made my choice, for my choice was not to be here with you physically. It was to be here with you in mind, body, and spirit in this particular way, for is that not still a special place to be, my dear one?

That we are apart but together and you can talk to me as if I am there with you and yet I am not – not in the usual sense of the word. And you may well miss me in your arms and you may well wonder what it is I would look like now and yet is it really as important as you thought it would be – for isn't this in fact what we are doing now?

So why do you need this physical form of myself so badly? It is a good question to ask all of your ladies, because the truth of this is that it is filling a hole that you need to unconditionally love and also be unconditionally loved.

And, yes, we all need this connection. Yet you women who have chosen this particular path of life and loss are the ones who are searching ever more deeply for the unconditional love that resides inside all of you anyway. It is just you cannot quite see it like that now.

For us 'babies' and us souls, who for whatever reason are holding back from coming fully into form, can offer you any amount of unconditional love whether we are with you physically or not. And so – do you see? – it is your own love and knowledge of this love that we can offer to you physically, or from afar, and indeed that is exactly the same kind of love.

For me and my re-joining of my soul once I had been released from the body. Oh, it was so utterly joyful and filled with light because I was finally free of the burden that we both have carried across lifetimes to begin this work of ours together.

I was also free to regain my whole soul, and I am telling you, there is no greater moment in your life when this happens, for it is a true celebration of what is home. Not to say that the moment before leaving the body is not a sad one, for it is always a joy to be in the arms of unconditional love in a mother's womb.

However, it is nothing in comparison to the explosion of light and joyfulness that comes from being free of that body, free of that world, and in my case, especially so when I was never meant to be coming into that world in the first place.

And this is why, even though I knew I would be creating hardship and heartache because of my choice, I also knew that if we did not go through with this plan as we had discussed on many an occasion in order to lift the world, then the hardship and heartache would indeed be far worse than you could ever have imagined, or can even imagine now.

For imagine that you are not doing this work. Imagine if you had never given yourself the opportunity to feel the love of a baby spirit for its mummy that you have brought through for them. Imagine never feeling that joy or seeing that joy on the face of the mums who are coming to you.

For it is all real and it is all happening and indeed must happen. You must get this book out into the world and enable the mums of these baby spirits here with me to somehow see the light of themselves so they can see the light of their babies here on earth and in spirit.

That is your job and your role and I will be here to ensure that it happens and for you to know it is not happening on its own. You will be guided, and I will be providing you with all that you need. Just as you trusted me before in many lifetimes since, when I felt you in my arms and I let you go, you too must now feel me in your arms and let me go to do what I need to do to make this happen.

I rejoiced for my soul and I celebrated with the many souls, with whom I am working, that our plan is in motion and the love that you needed to feel for you to go through with this, the love for yourself, was all in place and now we could take our part and our roles in this plan forward.

For I am not of the baby spirit world, I am of the higher realms, and it was never my intention to return to the baby spirit realm for I have no need to be there. I am no longer a baby wishing to be born into your world to sing and to dance and to learn and to love in this physical sense, for I am more than this now in these realms.

For now, my little love, it is time to focus on your worldly matters and your worldly story for it is getting in the way of our own particular story. And know that you are being guided and trust that we are here, I am here, to make sure, ensure, all is turning out as it should.

## Why babies choose not to stay

The above is an introduction to my and Rosa's journey together. My previous baby losses – all of whom I've discovered were girls – formed a part of this journey to awakening me onto my path, to awaken the energy of the Divine Mother which lies at the heart of my own Soul Plan.

So, what are the lessons from your own journeys to motherhood? They will, of course, be unique and you will find your answers if you choose to look. It has taken me years to understand my own journey with Rosa, for many reasons, but it doesn't have to be such a long, drawn-out exploration.

A beautiful soul who joined my closed Facebook group reached out to me via Messenger to share her guilt and anxiety around a termination she had had. Despite her choice to release her baby some years ago, and having four children and being a wonderful mum, she was finding it hard to forgive herself and felt huge amounts of guilt. She was very intuitive herself and knew the baby was a girl and the name Grace had come into her mind.

I knew the name was significant to her story and asked her to look up the meaning of Grace and what was going on in her life at that time. This amazing lady was in a very controlling and abusive relationship and she knew that having a baby would not be safe for either of them or her other children. She chose a termination, an extremely low point of her life, which was the catalyst for her to leave this unhealthy relationship.

Within a few messages backwards and forwards, this woman was able to see that her baby had never intended to come into the world at that time, that Grace the Soul loved her so much she had come in for just a short while to help her 'mum', through the divine law of Grace, move out of her unsafe relationship and start a new life.

This is the gift that our babies in spirit offer us. There are so many, many reasons why babies choose not to stay, or women find themselves in a situation where they have to make the choice no woman ever wants to make.

Also to know that your choice was an act of love. Love for yourself and your baby – and there is always, always a bigger picture.

As Rosa says about the circumstances of our story, and the body she chose to enter being one that wasn't medically considered viable, "For us, my darling Debra, your body and my body were perfect for the circumstance we chose because *we chose 'un-wholeness' for you to become whole*." I also asked her if she felt rejected by my choice:

**Me**: Did I reject you?

**Rosa**: On a soul level, no. On a human level, yes. Let's face it, you did not want me as I was not whole – no matter how much you dress it up. However, that was the 'whole' point, that you would feel this rejection and this loss and this yearning and this desperation for something different to have happened. Yet it did not and so it is to wholeness that you came back – making each other whole by accepting who we are on a soul level. A full circle if you like – my 'un-wholeness' in your eyes, drawing you towards 'wholeness'.

**Rosa's message below highlights some other reasons why babies may not choose to stay.**

Some babies are merely here for a short experience to know what it feels like to be in body and connect with their soul parents. They may only need a few short weeks to realise their potential on this earth and they may decide to come back or wait for another time and another set of circumstances.

These circumstances could be timing for them and their parents, particularly wealth or place of living, as each soul has a particular mission that they wish to experience and perhaps circumstances aren't quite right at this time.

Some babies may need to practice being in the density of the world before they can fully incarnate for a longer period of time. This doesn't mean that love isn't always around, because once you have touched the soul of your baby, they are forever with you – even if they decide to choose other parents at the time, they will always come back to you in one form or another.

Your spirit babies are your connection with the other worlds and many are simply here to let you know that – that there are other worlds, other imaginations, other lifetimes and other possibilities in your universe.

It is all about looking up to the sky and knowing where you came from, where you planned and plotted your life and all your experiences, including the connection with your spirit babies.

They are always with you, whether in person or in spirit, and may decide to come to you again in another form – as a niece or a nephew or a godchild. Do not fear, you will know who they are because you will have a spiritual connection with them.

Other babies simply change their minds as they review their life and decide it is not for them after all. This may be a particularly difficult challenge that they are guided to not go ahead with because circumstances aren't quite right.

It may also be the body they did not choose. For us, my darling Debra, your body and my body were perfect for the circumstance we chose because we chose 'un-wholeness' for you to become whole. Not all mums need to experience this to wake them up but you were particularly stubborn and blocked off.

And so our babies have choices and at some level, you have a choice too. Maybe you cannot offer what the baby needs at this time, and so you decide to let them go until you can manage this better and your own soul purpose in this relationship.

Maybe it is the wrong time for the child and they need to wait for someone else to pass until the time is right for them to appear. They can gain much knowledge and wisdom from their loved ones when they return to help them decide which path they wish to take and what to expect.

These loved ones may indeed become their guides and they need these guides, who are so connected to the family, in order to feel fully safe and informed before they enter.

Some babies arrive to highlight where healing is necessary within a relationship, the body or energy field that may be necessary for that mum or parent's soul growth.

Miscarriage is a joyful thing to experience in the end because it allows you stronger and better connection to All that is and to your spirit babies. It is sad on a human level of course because it is a difficult connection to break once on the earthly plane and it almost feels like being severed. But know the connection takes a different form after this, a more beautiful one. Since the need for connection is gone you allow each other the freedom to be as a whole, while remaining in contact and in each other's space and worlds.

So do not grieve for your little ones, as they enjoyed the best of times, and know they have experienced your love on many levels. It is just for now they choose to experience it in this way and not in a physical form.

If you could see all the baby souls with me now, you would not fret because they are all happy in their choices. They watch you from afar, waiting and wondering when they will be ready to come to you. Also watching and waiting for you to allow them to be ready for you.

For you mums it is the clearing of the womb, clearing of the space that will house your little souls so they know they are not coming in with fear, lack, or past lives that may throw them off their path, a path that is only love and bringing only their most special qualities down into the world at this time.

Many of them have seen and experienced much of what the earth has to offer and now wish to bring only joy and awakening to the process, for the earth is changing and these little souls of pure light are much needed.

There must be reassurance that their light will be able to shine brightly without the worries and woes of those they have chosen to join with. They need to be understood, to be the new wave of beings that bring light to the world, and if they are not given free rein to do so, their mission will be incomplete and their time not given to the best of what it could be.

This new wave of souls has a very special mission and therefore they must choose well their parents and their situations in order to do so. But they cannot do this alone and the mothers that they are seeking must first seek themselves and also wake up to the mission of light that they have willingly accepted in this lifetime.

Your job, dear Debra, is to bring light to the mums who live in the shadows of fear, for they are the carriers by which these little ones will bring light to the world.

Go well, with love. I am always with you. Rosa.

**A message from Rosa for those of you who have lost a child**

To those who fear they have lost their child and that they will never return, fear not, they are always here. They are waiting for the right time or the right body, or they are simply waiting to connect with you. They are never truly gone and those who choose not to come into form again at this time may well have had another service to provide, either for themselves or for you.

So listen well and know they are waiting here to reveal their answers if you so choose. It is not a big thing; it is not a scary thing. It is merely a thing that has happened in the great scheme of life that brings you back to your centre, back to your still point, back to your home, and to remember who you are and that nothing and no one truly ever dies.

It is with much love that I bring this message because it is not one of blame and nor is it one of judgement. It is one of love and enlightenment for the ways of the world. You are playing a much bigger game than you can ever imagine.

So, for now, simply imagine being with your little one. Being with your lost one for they are not lost. They are here and they are waiting, loving and sharing with you your dreams as well as their own from a place that may be unfamiliar to you but is no less real than the one you are currently seeing.

Know that this connection is possible. Know that they are real. Know that their stories and choices are real, and know that they are always by your side and you will be reunited at some point across the eons of time.

For they have chosen you to feel them in your space and perhaps they chose not to stay in your space for as long as you'd hoped. However, it is a space that is never-ending and a love that is never dying and you will know who they are when you meet again, whether it is in this lifetime or the next.

It is not the end, it is never the end, and I live to tell the tale of many lives and many people and now I am here to share and to tell of the many new stories that are coming, and the many new ways of how we all look at the world.

And I am with you. For always. And sending so much love to all of you who are grieving and all of you in pain and all of you who are waiting. For there is no greater prize than to love yourself amid it all. And I am here to beam that love down to you so you can feel it for yourselves, for you are the key that can unlock it not only for yourselves but also for your babies here and in form and indeed the whole world.

And it is with these words that I leave you now. Feel this love that I offer, receive it, for it is yours and yours alone. It is time to acknowledge this truth of yourselves, that you are indeed the love and it is the love that unites and reunites.

Go well, my little ones, my lost ones, my special ones, for the light is coming to you. Of that do not doubt.

And so it is.

Knowing the answer to your question of 'why did this happen?' from a bigger picture perspective and your spirit baby's perspective, is hugely healing and comforting. However, the feelings that baby loss brings up and how you're thinking about yourself because of it must also be explored. Our human selves, physical body, thoughts and emotions, need to be given space to catch up with the spiritual knowing. I buried my emotions after my losses, but just because I chose not to see and feel them, didn't mean they were no longer there. Much of it was holding me back from other opportunities and being who I truly am.

We hold this pain in our cellular memory, mental and emotional bodies. They were likely there long before your loss, it's your loss that has brought them to the surface so you have the opportunity to release and transform them. Your life doesn't have to be dictated by your experience. I know it may not feel like it right now, but you can and will move through the confusion and hurt to a deeper understanding and find peace within it and yourself. If you have experienced baby loss, any loss, this is a trauma. And allowing yourself to heal and find resolution allows you to come out of trauma and feeling stuck in the moment of it. We explore this further in the following chapters.

For now, please hold onto Rosa's words as you allow yourself to feel your grief. Writing down how you feel, and what you're making your feelings mean about you and for you, is such a cathartic process. A deep step into freeing yourself from pain and into more knowing of who you are. I cover the experience of termination further on in the book, but whilst we are looking at baby loss, I wanted to make a special mention for those of you who have experienced loss at the very late stages of pregnancy. What we call stillbirth and what the spirit baby realm refers to as non-earth birth.

## Still birth – or non-earth birth as the babies describe it

I have supported women who have experienced this level of loss, and as with any loss, it is not something you 'get over' to move on with your life. It is an experience you can learn to honour and live with. It is one you can live with more peacefully, the more you are able to explore, transform and ease your thoughts and emotions around your loss; the more you connect with yourself and your angel baby to understand the bigger picture.

It is not an experience that is spoken about freely, which can further add to the trauma. Support, understanding, and kindness are, of course, key for the parents. Just as I was finishing writing this book there were a lot of blocks to actually birthing it and I decided it was time to explore my own healing around my now eight-year-old Samuel's conception and birth.

In the ninth and final session with the gorgeous Hazel Boylan, a fellow author and birth matrix practitioner, I was finally at the point of reimagining Samuel's birth when I felt this huge anxiety. I had cleared so many layers by now I was a bit exasperated as to what else could possibly be holding me back from the final birthing stages! We followed the energy of worry and I was taken to a memory of being a baby who chose not to stay at the last moment.

The anxiety I felt was that if I had made that decision as a baby myself at one point in time, what was to stop my children from making that same choice? What if my baby chose not to stay at or after the moment of birth? I transformed the energy and the learning from it was huge. It was all part of my training over many lifetimes with Rosa to experience all aspects of coming into life. As my other lifetime baby self, I was able to sense the unconditional love I had for my mother then, the comfort I offered her from a non-physical place that she wasn't aware of.

I know with a full heart your babies love you and this doesn't change whether they are with you physically or not. They have a choice and it is nothing to do with whether you are good enough or not.

As with all of life, the reasons for a baby choosing not to be born here are as unique as you and they are. Some of the reasons are beyond our imaginations of just how big the bigger picture is, including one such incredible high-born soul whose energy of love is impossible to put into words and rarely felt here on earth. Her short earth role was to gather as much information as possible as to what life was like in the womb of her beautiful mum in order to guide and teach future souls of an extremely high vibration, highly evolved, considering coming to earth, to help them prepare for life on earth. Truly a new generation of new earth souls and energy coming into the planet.

Your babies are not helpless beings. They are powerfully loving souls with a background and mission of their own. And it may or may not ease your pain right now to know about stories such as this, and you may also wonder, why you? Please know that you do hold the answers to your questions when you're ready to find them and find who you are within it all. At a soul level, the depth of the love you offer and are, the connection you have with this soul, enabled your baby soul the opportunity to experience life here, to feel your love, if only from the safety of your womb. There is nothing you did or didn't do other than show up as one of the bravest, most courageous and strong women of the world, and at some point, your experience of such pain, and why you were the one to feel it, will become clear.

Rosa has some more words to add that you may or may not wish to read right now, depending on where you are on your healing journey. I fully appreciate that the human experience can far outweigh any sense of comfort offered by a spiritual context. Holding you all in love, the words below are for when and if you feel ready.

## Rosa on non-earth births

I will do my best, darling Debra, to explain in as few words as possible the experience that you know as stillbirth. Even the very name you have given this experience sends shock waves throughout the universe. For there is no such thing as a stillbirth in our realms. For if a soul chooses to remain behind in a physical body then the birth is very much of and in the earth. And if a soul chooses to leave its body behind, then there is a birth back into and of the higher realms and dimensions whichever way and in whichever place a soul wishes to travel.

Yet this does not answer your question and neither does it lift any of the plight or the grief from the womb, hearts and souls of the women and their men who have been through this grievous loss of love. For this is most certainly what it feels like. A loss of love, life, kindness, and a loss of self, not to mention a most grievous loss, that of trust. Trust in one's body, trusting one's baby, and – yes – trusting one's universe. It is in this moment that it must feel like the universe has crumbled and that there is no more.

Yet somehow life carries on, love carries on. And somehow trust carries on in some quarters of your life. How can this be so when such a devastating blow has been dealt that you feel you will never, and perhaps even wish to never, recover from?

There are also many other reasons for baby souls to choose to remain in the life beyond life. Perhaps one of these reasons is indeed to bridge the gap between heaven and earth. For every incidence of rebirth, stillbirth as you call it, a non-earth birth as we know it, is as unique to each person, as each person is unique.

For many, this experience will be the catalyst which wakes them up to grief, wakes them up to loss, and ultimately wakes them up to the connection that comes even through loss, that in some way can help a deeper healing process, which is necessary and was necessary for that soul.

Often it is the child who simply wishes to experience life upon this earth from the safety of its mother's womb. To remember and to awaken it to times gone past and times that may still come in another time and place when that soul feels comfortable enough and ready to do so. Often there are karmic ties between these children and their parents, and their love of life and loss is playing out here unbeknownst to them.

Harder for you to understand, and yet of no less love from the perspective of the souls who wished not to be birthed into this plane of density that is the earth, are those disgruntled souls who manage to find their way into the light and the love of an adoring parent. These can be hurting souls and vulnerable souls and we are asking you to firstly forgive yourselves, for you too knew on some level what this soul was needing from you and you were willing to give the soul and love the soul into being with a love and a force so strong that their past hurts and pains would simply disappear as if in an instant.

Yet for many, this is not the case and their pains do not disappear. Only the bravest and most open-hearted women will take on, and give a chance to love such a soul. Only the bravest and most open-hearted are prepared to risk the damage to their own soul if there is a turnaround in events and this young soul cannot yet see a way through the hurt they are in, and so must return to the light once again to reflect on and review the life and the lives they have had. They need further healing before once again landing upon the earth and into the arms of the love of their mothers.

And they will do so when it is their time. So please do forgive them. For they too are trying to heal their own pain. It is our heartfelt wish that you give these souls another chance and give these souls another love of life so they too can truly heal and be on their way to being a spreader of the love that is held by the mothers they choose now, and not the spreader of the pain from the mothers that have so often gone before them, who too were in very deep pain.

This is the way of the souls, and this is the way of the universe, expressing itself as all things and in all ways, in pain, loss and heartache and, sadly, tragedy. In all those expressions of pain that are seen in order to only show up the absolute opposite of this pain, which is of course love.

So it is this love of life, which often dies alongside the death of hope that comes from a non-birth onto the earth, which is also a purveyor and a carrier of the potential for true rebirth. A rebirth into the light of that soul who has chosen to remain above for now and a rebirth of a life imagined by the chosen parents of that soul.

For it is only to this life that we can choose to rediscover life in this moment.

Sending love to all of you brave and courageous woman and men as you navigate into a life you had not imagined and may this unfold now with many blessings.

# Chapter 4
## Who is Rosa?
## Have you lived previous lifetimes with your children and future children?

To me, Rosa is the baby I released. Our experience together led to the light in me being switched off for a while, only to be switched back on even brighter than I could ever have imagined possible. But as I have grown into myself and discovered more and more of who I am, and of the energy that I carry out into the world, I am always asking Rosa – who are you?

Before I was channelling and connecting with her energy, I met with some incredibly gifted mediums – all of whom said their own guides were telling them that Rosa was a very high vibration soul from the higher realms, but they couldn't connect with her themselves.

I turned again to the name that had popped into my head, long before I even knew or at least acknowledged that I was able to communicate with spirit – the spirit I had named as Rosa Mai Kilby. Now, as a Soul Plan Reader, I am aware of how vital our names are – they are like a secret code to who we are. Your name sets the intention for your life experiences. Your full birth name, whether adopted or changed for whatever reason, on the whole, remains your dominant vibration. Nicknames, married names, bring in new energies, which bring in new experiences, but your original name sets the scene. Each letter has a unique sound vibration that interacts with the universal energies – your name connects you to the people, opportunities and situations which will enable you to fulfil the call from your soul to achieve your soul purpose.

Your name is how you introduce yourself to the world, to people, and there is a powerful energy released each time you say your name or your name is called. The way we are given our names varies across cultures. As with everything, there is a much bigger picture as to who or how we end up with our names, but I believe there is no such thing as an accident. Whoever names you is acting as a channel of the intention and your name is fundamental to your relationship with the world. I have read and shared the Soul Plan of many clients whose birth certificates had a spelling 'mistake', or those who are adopted and their birth name is different from their current passport or official name now. It never ceases to amaze me how they resonate more with the energies, the challenges, the gifts, and the goals of their original birth name than with the name they go by now.

There is the meaning of your name that you can check on many websites, and there is also a history that follows. Your name offers a clue to your lineage as well as your purpose. It's a really interesting exercise to explore your name meaning more deeply, and if you set the intention of 'knowing' when you do this, a little spark of recognition will be lit.

The root of Debra, or Deborah, in Hebrew comes from the root 'to speak or to pronounce'. Deborah was also a war leader and prophetess. I'm not claiming to be a prophetess by any stretch, but the soul plan messages that come through aren't snapshot psychic readings but lifelong messages that – some of the receivers of them have said – are prophetic. The more they read them over time, the more they understand and see them happening. Rosa's vision for our lives and the earth can certainly fall within this bracket.

My middle name is Mary. It's my mum's middle name and the name of my grandmother on my dad's side. But I never liked it for myself. I grimaced every time I had to say it. It's old fashioned and made me think of religion, which I was never that impressed with as a child. I didn't want to 'own' that name. The irony is that I now channel the energies of Mother Mary and Mary Magdalene, as well as Isis and Kali, among other beings, who represent the Divine Mother energy. It is this energy of the Divine Mother that lies at the heart of my own Soul Plan, my life-purpose energy – the energy that I'm here to live my fullest potential from. I feel I'm owning this name more and more; we grow into our names, as we grow into our soul's plan.

For Rosa, the rose flower is the highest vibration flower on the planet – hugely healing for the heart. It is a flower that is given as an indication of love and one that asks you to open your heart to receive love.

It is also a flower that helps you to heal wounds of the past. When we have been through painful experiences such as the loss of a loved one or being hurt by the words or actions of somebody close to us, we can carry that hurt in our hearts, leaving blockages in our heart chakra. Bringing the energy of the rose into our heart space helps us to heal and melt away these wounds so we can move forward in our lives, being open to receiving more love.

The rose has been the sacred symbol of many important goddesses associated with love, including Ishtar, Aphrodite, Isis, and Mother Mary, who is also known as the Mystic Rose, the rose without thorns, representing original, uncorrupted purity, as well as a vital creative principle. It is a name that represents the Divine Mother energy and is a heart-opening name, and that is certainly what Rosa's and my experience together brought about in me. The many connections to the Divine Mother energy can send my head spinning as to who Rosa is and the nature of our connection.

The name Mai is derived from Mary, my own middle name and, of course, the name of the Divine Mother in the Roman Catholic tradition. The synchronicities keep on coming – I had no idea of the depth of name readings and the importance of the name Rosa had given me to name her at her funeral.

The name Rosa Mai Kilby holds the energies of speech and communication – speaking a message clearly and confidently and sharing it out – as well as the energy of unity and magnetism – bringing like-minded people together to bring about change. Her name also holds the energy of the Divine Mother – unconditional love. At the heart of this name, the life purpose energy is that of earth, emotions, and society – literally bringing a message down from above.

I can't tell you how in awe I was when my friend and fellow Soul Plan Reader, Karen Goodson, suggested I take a look at the Soul Plan energies of Rosa's name whilst writing this book. A name I 'heard' a few weeks after releasing Rosa.

The Soul Plan system is a new interpretation of an ancient system of life purpose analysis, channelled by Blue Marsden. It works on the conscious and unconscious levels, revealing the energies in your soul's plan that bring your challenges to the fore, your gifts that help you move through your challenges to reach your goals, and ultimately your life purpose energy – your highest potential in this lifetime.

The Soul Plan system created by Blue Marsden never ceases to amaze me or the people who come for a reading – they finally feel seen. And here I was seeing Rosa's Soul Plan now coming to life before my very eyes. Her life purpose of bringing spiritual messages down to earth is playing out – even though she is not physically here – because her messages are coming through me.

But every time I asked Rosa who she was, I didn't receive a reply. Until one day the following message came through. I hope it helps you to know that you and your babies, whether here with you, or on earth, have not only chosen to be together in this lifetime, but have very likely been with you in many other lifetimes too.

**Who is Rosa?**

> **Me**: Who are you?
>
> **Rosa**: Who is anyone? We are all and everything of the all and everything. We are a part of the trees and the flowers, the earth and the seas. Have you not sensed this yet? For this is where we are all heading, to know completely and fully that we are not at all separate from anything or anyone.
>
> However, if you are asking, 'who have I been?', 'what have I done?', then this is a very different question and one that may take some time to answer, seeing as I have lived many lives, 3,160 to be precise. And in those times I have been many people and many things.
>
> I'm guessing the ones you would like to know about are the ones pertaining to our story and our book. And this too is hard to whittle down and separate, as we have been together for so many of these lives.

Open up to hear the ones that you wish to hear. Trust that my words are coming to you and through you, and relax into the energy of my mind as it was, and not yours as it is now. Relax, relax, relax and let go and allow all the images and pieces of the puzzle to come through.

## Aspects of Rosa – the warrior princess

So you are seeing now the image of a warrior princess in high battle taking her sword out to fight those who have invaded our land. I was not one for sitting around dawdling and allowing things to happen. I had stuff to be doing, principles to uphold, and life and love and land to battle for, and battle I did.

As a woman in the exact tunic you are seeing now, I was a Christian, but not in the sense that you have of Christianity. The helmet is reminiscent of the time. I was a woman and a warrior, and that was quite unusual for that time, but I managed to impress upon people that I had every right to fight for my land, the same as anyone else. And with no babies and no husband, I felt my purpose was to do just that.

And I did it well. I was held in high regard for the battles I fought, like a gladiator. I was all about protecting the faith, protecting the faith of myself, my God and my Nero* and to that end, nothing else came into it.

I was brainwashed into believing that he, and his and my beliefs, were all and everything. So when I say a Christian, it is in this sense, that I was right and everyone else was wrong, that I was coming from. That was the belief system I was in.

It was only when I came with child that my mindset changed entirely. This child who gazed at me with such trust and perfection, inviting me to love, to cherish and to nurture; to put aside my anger and my hatred and my need to impress. It is then, in that moment, that I became a woman. A woman in the sense that all my warrior power and battles, and the striving of being noticed by my Nero, were suddenly changed and my focus widened to what was really possible if one was just able to love. To love unconditionally, without right or wrong, or without battling or striving for it, or trying to impress; simply to gaze upon love with innocent eyes and that trusting knowledge of you are the one to hold, help, feed, provide, and to love that little being.

This is what our children offer us, an entirely different perspective on life. A life that is not about battle, a life that is not about being the best. A life that is not about prowess and doing things for others in the hope of being someone. For these little beings are already someone – someone who has not done anything in the world as yet, and yet is loved unconditionally for that.

It is to this state of knowledge, that we have to do nothing, nothing at all to be loved, for we are all loved, as these babies are loved the minute they arrive and look into our eyes with such adoration and with such knowing that they are all they need to be.

This is what our babies tell us and this is what our babies teach us, remind us: that we do not need to be anything, to prove anything, to do anything to be loved, for we are already loved. It is this state of knowingness that our readers will be reminded of and taken back to. Their first moments of unconditional love on this planet, which for many lasted no more than a few seconds. However, a few seconds is all it takes to know the true beauty of who you are in all your naked glory, without a whim or a care in the world.

You have come from God and there is no reason to expect anything other than the same world from which you have just arrived. However, for many that world soon changes and our battles begin. My point for this story though, is that everything changes once we remember the love that we are and the love we have come from. We are love, and with this force, there is no need for any other force. No need to force love, to force wisdom, to force ourselves, or others. There is no force necessary at all, for we are taken back to that very first state of love, and with these words, so it is.

\* When I double-checked with Rosa about the name, Nero, and whom she was referring to, the answer that came was: "Nero is the name of the man I was in love with, not the man of your tales but of mine. He is the Nero of your dreams and your nightmares. The one who came and saw and conquered, but not in the life of the lands and the people, but in the heart and mind of myself, for he was the man who couldn't abide the love of any women, and so I became the man in the woman in order for him to be loved by me and for me. I knew no other way back then of pleasing people, least of all myself. And so this is my Nero, my opposite of love, in the twisted way I believed love to be at that time."

I am still not clear in my human mind about this answer of Rosa's. I get the sense that she doesn't mean Nero, the corrupt, cruel Roman emperor, but a man who represented the unsavoury Nero-type energy.

## Aspects of Rosa – the midwife

My second story I wish to share, in order for you to gain a perspective on who I am in terms of your human way of looking at life, is the life I spent as a midwife. Your midwife in fact, my dear. Not in this lifetime, but another not so long ago.

You can see the dress and imagine the time it was then, for again it was conflict time and war raged around us. No sooner were you born, than you died in my arms amid the blood and carnage of that tent that day, out in a field of France.

I had no idea who you were, and yet I was touched beyond misery of the misery of your mother as you lay in her arms sleeping, unable to cope with the violence that surrounded you, with the turmoil of the world and the depths of human depravity that you witnessed as you came into this world.

And so you chose to leave, to come back another time when more peace reigned, and you were able to deal better with the ways of the world. It was simply not the right time.

But your poor mother was inconsolable and blamed herself for being in this part of the world and not listening to her intuition to leave this land when she had the chance. And now she had lost you, unable to see that it was you who had left her for the greater good and not she who was in the wrong and who had made that choice, but you.

And we became great friends, your mother and I, in that lifetime. And as her own life dwindled away, bereft of the daughter she had so prayed for, we made a promise to each other to find you on the other side and to all reunite together once again.

And that we did, my little one, for of course, we had known each other many times before and this was yet another re-enactment of the many scenarios we played out together, practising our lives, learning our lessons, growing in our love and understanding of love and life and what was part of that.

Our latest reincarnation together has been this one, in which the roles were reversed. And no, I wasn't your midwife this time, but the baby who was to make that choice, and for you to be the mother who witnessed and experienced the consequences of that choice. That choice of a baby who was not ready, not willing, not able to make it through into the chaos of this physical world. For you to be the mother left behind, with all the grief and recrimination, the failure and the pain, that this loss of a baby brings about.

You have done well, my little one, for you have turned this story of yours around now. Made up your lessons in love and letting go and allowing of free choice, no matter how impossibly difficult that seems to many.

And yet you did, and here you are now, sharing this choice from both the perspective of the baby you once were, who chose not to stay, but also the perspective of the mother who had to let her baby go, because at some level, some very deep knowing, you knew this was the choice of your baby – my choice.

My choice not to stay in the body that was formed. And so you had to let me go and this is your karma, and this is our karma and through healing our old wounds of helplessness and despair, ineffectiveness and failures, love and loss, do you see now we are able to reach out to other women with a depth of understanding that would never be, if we hadn't lived these often painful lives together?

It has not all been about the pain. But also about the love, for in my last story, it was I who held you as you came into the world and left, but previous to that it was you who held me. You held me on the battlefield, you held me in the trenches of war, you held me in your arms as the ever-loving soul you are and you held me in my light when I was shining down at you from afar.

My beautiful, we have been on many journeys together and you and I have played many roles. This latest role is all but the next step in our journey, and one which we both agreed would not only complete the karma in order for you to shine, but also complete the cycle of life and lives we have known together.

My journey on earth for the time being, and perhaps always, has come to an end as I take my other duties and responsibilities of love from on high. Not on high as in above you, but on high as another level; whereas you, brave soul, have offered yourself to the world again, despite the continuing chaos, knowing of the role you are to play in bringing about a New Earth, a new dimension to the reality we currently see, and of lifting the world yet again into a new age.

My role from on high is to be your guide and be your mentor and shine down my love for you to be the open spirit and channel we see today.

One who will bring back that knowing of love in its purest form for people to remember, and see, as I did on the birth of my own baby, that love resides within. It is expected, it is a done deal, it is a knowing and it is a right and no amount of parenting will ever change the fact that our babies are pure love.

It is with this love now that they are asking to come down onto earth. They will not come until they see that the greatness and pure love that they are is recognised. So to all parents who are reading this book, this book of love, who are waiting for their babies to arrive, or for their babies in spirit who they may feel are lost to them, know that they are not lost, but instead waiting here, with me, to be honoured for the true beings they are, with a history and a mission and a plan and an expectation of love that knows no bounds.

They will not and cannot get through the web of density into the real world of you, unless they know their needs are in place and that their plans are accepted in full. This is not a scary thing. This is not a big thing. This is not a worrying thing or a threat. It is a simple fact that humans now must know that the love that their babies carry for them is met by the love of yourselves. That we all know that moment of arrival as a whole being, with plans and dreams and ambitions and quirks, that has been hard fought for over many centuries, is allowed to be just that.

Whole and pure and simply them, in all their glory and with all their personality intact, and unable to be moulded into something they are not. Can we do this for our children? Our children of light? For they are coming and for many, their wait is over and so we must be ready for them. Ready to receive them from a place of our own high vibration in order that they, and we, can be the full expression of ourselves as spirits in human form.

As for me, I am, too, watching and waiting and playing and

loving your babies, willing and urging you with so much love to connect with yourselves and connect with us, so that you know we are coming to you, when the time is right, and you are able to hold us in that pure love that each and every one of us desire and deserve, and are.

So, be at one with your own light. Be at one with your own dreams and desires, not from a place of fear or unworthiness, but from a place of sheer power and knowing who you are and what you are, so in turn, you can recognise your own babies, in whichever way they come to you, as powerful, beautiful souls in their own right, with their own powers and histories.

It is with so much love that I greet you all in this way and for you to hear my words from a place of so much wonder and light that is filled with special souls, your souls, who are waiting and watching with excitement and hope and love that you will be the ones who are helping them to create a New Earth.

See them, feel them, hear them, and invite them into your lives so they can travel through the mists of time, travel through the web of density that currently surrounds them, and greet you in mind, body, and spirit, as is their wish.

Go well, my mothers and fathers, and find your light. For within it you will find the light of your next aspect of soul. And so it is. With my blessings and unconditional love that I rain down on you.

Forever and for always. In love.

Rosa

As I was re-reading and editing this section of the book, I knew I was receiving more messages about who Rosa is, but I was too close and in too much resistance to hearing the answer to get a clear sense for myself without thinking I was making it up.

It was another gifted and gorgeous friend, Olwen Jennings, who channels her guides – think the UK version of Abraham Hicks – whom I turned to. I knew I was getting closer and closer to accepting something about myself and about Rosa. Olwen's guides – who call themselves the Meta-Collective – said they were being shown an image of a womb, the womb of Mother Mary. Rosa is an aspect of, the energy of, or holds the energy of, the Divine Mother who represents the womb. Woah, I know, I was already freaking out by this stage myself! Stay with me, it will become clearer.

When I mention names such as Mother Mary, it's easier for our conscious minds to imagine an actual person and form. It's also easy to go straight to the stories we've been told about her. Maybe it's time to question those stories, who told them and why? Is this their truth or hers? One day I may be writing a story of Mary from her own perspective. How powerful this would be.

Energy is expansive and everywhere and not confined to a form as we see it. You are in form, in your body, but your energy isn't confined to your body, it's vast and expansive. Mother Mary is a name we put to an energy, a consciousness, to make it easier to comprehend in our human mind. The energy of Mother Mary brings up feelings of being held, loved, safe, that everything is going to be okay. She also brings in the energy of possibility, miracles, hope, self-love, and empowerment. There are so many examples of her image appearing at various times across the world, at seemingly desperate times, helping to uplift communities. Energy knows no time and space, it is not bound by anything, it is limitless. Mother Mary was a woman who brought in this consciousness that we can all access if we choose.

She is, of course, also an energy that births the light. You and your babies all bring your energy, new consciousness to this planet. You are the light and are birthers of light. The energy of Mother Mary is always with me and with the women I work with helping you to know this is who you are. Holding you and your babies in love so that you can come together if and when the time is right. Without women, there is no light, there is no life being birthed. Can you feel how important that makes you? How powerful you are? Take a moment to recognise where you feel unimportant, breathe into this energy whilst repeating in your mind: I am a birther of light. Feel this energy change.

# Chapter 5
## Sacred Conception
### Behind the scenes of spirit baby to earth baby

As women, as mums, or mums who have lost babies, or mums who are waiting for their babies to arrive, we know deep, deep inside our hearts that our babies are unique, special little beings in their own right. But often this point is missed when we're trying to get pregnant, and especially so if part of our journey to motherhood is through a more medical route.

Getting pregnant is not simply a physical act. You are creating life. You are not only making a baby, you are birthing new life, a new consciousness into the world. You are inviting another beautiful soul into your lives, a soul with their own mission, their own life path, their own challenges, gifts and goals, a soul who has likely lived many lives before, a soul you have likely lived with many times before. And I, as a therapist, spiritual counsellor and spirit baby communicator – and Rosa – am asking you to recognise this.

We are powerful spiritual beings living in a physical human body. Everything we do, from washing the dishes to making love, is spiritual because that is who we are. We are made of love; we are love. This is what I mean when I talk about sacred conception. You are honouring your own soul and that of your baby or future baby. Knowing this brings a whole new level of meaning to the phrase 'making love'. By creating life, you are making love. By making love, you are creating life.

This is the same for mums whose babies will come to them through IVF and other medical procedures. Scientifically, there is a spark of light, a burst of energy that takes place as an embryo and sperm meet outside of the womb and a connection is made. A team from Northwestern University filmed the moment the egg and sperm meet and captured the mini firework display created as the zinc stored in the egg released for up to two hours after fertilisation.

This spark of life can be explained by the levels of zinc and various chemical reactions in a healthy egg and is, of course, controversial, sparking arguments for both pro-life and pro-choice about the efficacy of the experiment itself and what it means. I'm clearly not a scientist and hold no judgement on people's choices or beliefs either way, however, I've been honoured to be shown this beautiful event happening for my clients meeting their babies through IVF and egg donation – both occasions where egg and sperm have already met before physically settling into their new home of the womb and even before I've met the client. For me, I see it as a beautiful confirmation of a pregnancy. I've even witnessed a soul coming in before egg and sperm have met. The soul coming into the energy of their future mum, getting a sense of their mum's energy whilst waiting for the body. Whether they stay or come in and out until the physical process aligns, I don't know. But pregnancy has followed.

So, as is perhaps perfectly fitting, the moment of a soul coming in remains a mystery, at least to me for now. A miracle, that neither science nor anyone perhaps can explain. There are many psychics and channels, many articles around this subject which vary from life coming in at conception or not coming in until birth and not fully coming in until teenage years, and I'm happy to hold my hands up and say I don't know. All I know is what I've been shown, which is very different each time. Perhaps like each of us, this process is unique to each person and soul.

Whatever the miracle energy that allows life, your babies have a choice in this. I also believe that even if you are not physically 'making love' to create life, you are still making 'love', love being the essence and being of you and your baby and creating life. Spirit babies know exactly what they are doing and what needs to be done, and if they choose to come in, and if the stage is set, then they will come.

Of course, all conception is sacred, but have you ever wondered what is happening beyond the physical conception? The bigger, bigger picture really is way too big for us to even imagine.

**Here is a little insight from Rosa:**

Conception is often thought of as a purely physical act

of lovemaking at the right time, the right place, the right egg and the right sperm and the right bodies to make this happen. However, can you consider that there is perhaps something else going on around this sacred act? That this moment of conception is a meeting of heaven and earth? That this conception is one of spirit meeting spirit on this earthly plane and joining together as one in order for much greater things to happen?

Is it possible that, as this sperm meets this egg, there is so much more to be seen in the ripples of the whole universe? That it is not just between one man and one woman but it is indeed the whole universe in action? An action that will have momentous effects in the world, effects that this little one will have on the people they meet, the things they do, their energy that they share with the world, and their mission in this life?

Is it possible that conception is much, much more than a simple act of lovemaking, but is indeed a world changer, a universe mover, an embodiment of life itself, as the creators and co-creators of life choose to make it this moment, in this time and space and in this body and in this part of the world to come into form?

Do you think this is an accident? Do you think this life, this moment, has no further repercussions in the world than those for the parents and its family?

I think you know the answer to this for do you not recognise the impact that you have had in the world? The people you have met, touched, and changed in either kindness or in other ways? The changes you have made to yourself, and to and for others, which in turn have changed lives down the line?

And so, you see, this beautiful act of creation is not a simple physical act. It is a moment, yet another moment, in the awakening and the changing of the world itself as another new soul arrives to add their very unique flavour and sounds to the vibration and upliftment of the world.

It is this jigsaw of life coming together and apart, each forming a perfect piece in a perfect puzzle. And so it is that these precious souls here in spirit do choose to come together at a certain time and at a certain place and at a certain moment in order to fulfil and fill this world with life and all of life.

For those for whom conception has not yet come, do not fear and do not worry for there is always something bigger to be found here on this journey.

For those for whom conception was just this moment in time and you feel that this moment did not affect the future as I have spoken of above, yet again, do not fear, for this moment of conception, no matter how, when, for whom or for how long, truly does shift and change the sands of time in your own world and beyond.

So please, we ask you to acknowledge these brave spirits who are willing to come to spread life with you and add their flavour to the world, no matter for how long this may be. To acknowledge those spirits who choose to enable this moment of creation to happen, to create the energy of life in whichever way that may be.

For whatever you may think and feel about life, it is indeed life you have chosen and it is indeed life that these baby spirits are seeking. It is then up to you which picture of life you choose to present to them.


## Natasha's story

Two years ago, my beautiful friend, Natasha, who has allowed me to share her story here, was a single mum, hiding away from the world. A very difficult start to life from her birth, a long-term and difficult relationship in her teens to thirties, left her feeling all sorts of helpless and, mostly, shame.

It was a burden that wasn't hers to carry but left her feeling worthless and undeserving of love. Less than two years ago, our paths crossed as neighbours. Natasha had begun embracing the bigger picture – her 'why'. But after a 'chance' meeting at a moment of vulnerability, leading to a cup of tea at my house, a chat and a sprinkle of magic – to cut a long story short – Natasha allowed herself to live as her 'self', and own her story, and not be beholden to it or trapped by it.

Within a few short months, synchronicity after synchronicity brought Natasha and her now partner, Adrian, together – brought two families together and created a new one, with little Zen the latest addition. It was a life that had seemed so out of reach only a short time before.

I have asked Natasha to write about her experience of conscious conception and the moment she knew the soul we now know as Zen chose to commit to this physical world.

## Natasha recollects the conception moment

In the spring of May 2016, I sat alone, single, mostly lonely, and having resigned myself that this would be my life for the next sixty years; the idea of a conscious conception was as far away as the stars. Fast-forward to 27 May 2018 and the stars not only came to me, so close that I could touch and feel them, but they aligned in a way that is almost indescribable. Nevertheless, I will attempt to describe my experience, a real experience, (my nine-month-old son, Zen, is the proof that it was very real) a profound experience, my first experience – and who knows? – maybe my last experience.

It was a Sunday evening. It wasn't planned. If it had been, it would have been the perfect plan, but I won't take credit for how the event, or series of events, unravelled. You could say it was ordained and we were meant to be there, because although there was zero planning – everything, every detail, every motion – fell into place. It was like it had been rehearsed over and over again and then the event went according to plan. It was pure perfection. If you had asked my partner, Adrian, and me to repeat it – I can assure you – we couldn't have. However, on this one night we were on top form, and not just in a physical sense. In fact, I believe the physicality of that night was purely to serve the spirituality of that night – the physical, the spiritual, working together in a perfect symbiotic relationship.

Of course, it wasn't the first time Adrian and I had made love, and of course, we had enjoyed beautiful interactions many times before this one night. We hadn't done anything different. We hadn't discussed it – there was nothing to discuss. But on this one night, there was something different in the ether. The elements were aligning to create magic. I say magic because what happened that night was bigger than myself and my partner; it was beyond us. However, we acknowledge that without us, and the choices we made then, it would not have been possible. Hence all the elements, both known and unknown, were in perfect harmony and working with perfect precision.

The first element is that Adrian and I love each other and, as nauseating as it may sound, from our love springs forth wanting, fancying, appreciating, and all the other things love should conjure. There were no expectations of anything. We felt equally free to be, to fall into love and to make love. Of course, this can happen on any day and has happened many times before between us, but for this night we needed the other elements to be available and willing.

The second element was we felt drawn to play background music: 528Hz Open Heart Chakra, Love frequency, heart chakra activation and love. 528HZ is a beautiful frequency, and once you understand frequency in the maintaining and creation of life, on reflection, it makes sense.

Open heart chakra, love frequency and the activation of such speaks for itself – it was clear that our love hearts were both activated – in fact, we were bursting at the seams (in a metaphysical sense). I quickly realised something magical was happening, because not only was I experiencing an almost out-of-body experience (bear with me, as mentioned, it's difficult to describe), but tears were flowing from my eyes.

We have all heard that old cliché, 'the room spun'. Let me tell you, the cliché on this night was so real, more real than real life. The room did spin, and the colours that accompanied the spinning were breathtaking, smoky swirls of pinks, purples and violets – pastel colours working in perfect time. The 528Hz – it took me away. We were not engaged in a physical act, and even though I knew it at the time, my partner confirmed to me afterwards that he experienced the exact same feelings I experienced at the exact same time. And that is why my tears flowed – for I was experiencing beauty and magic as I had never experienced before.

The moment lasted an age, and during it, I heard myself say three times, "I receive you." "I receive you." "I receive you!" Where that came from and why I said it I could not begin to tell you. Had I been conscious of my thoughts and words I can assure you I may have thought it but would not have uttered them – not least because if I had a chance to think about it, I would have been sure my partner would have thought, "What is she on?!" But I was engaged with my partner in the highest level of trust and spirituality and it felt okay to be as vulnerable as I was in that moment. It was as though we had formed the DNA of what was to come. Literally, if I had closed my eyes I would have seen code becoming form and form becoming life. Our energy had created the energy that waited to be created.

After the event, the room spun out and my partner and I must have held each other tenderly for about half an hour. And it was then I said to him with a certainty that was more certain than certain, "You know we just created a baby, right!" He replied, "I know we did!" with the same certainty. When I asked him what he had experienced, he said it was like a psychedelic trip without the psychedelics – magical, blissful, emotional, and beautiful. And nine months later to the day, our son, Zen, was born. He will always be a reminder of our magic, the magic we created. On reflection, we as humans are indeed capable of such love when we surrender ourselves, and free ourselves from our egos. If we do this, nothing is promised, but everything is possible.

Zen was very much willing and wanting to share his thoughts and energy throughout the pregnancy. He even joined me on a Divine Feminine retreat I was running – but that's another story! Now he's here in the flesh, what a very special little dude he is, with a very special mum and dad who both embraced their own spiritual connection with themselves, each other, and Zen. Who I believe orchestrated the whole thing.

Just beautiful.

What is also beautiful is that before Natasha shared her story with me, I was guided to record a meditation to Meet your Spirit Baby for a programme of conscious conception run by the heart living and loving organisation that is Motherheart.org. The meditation guides women up into the spirit baby realm, and what do they find there? A vortex of colourful, swirling love. A coincidence and confirmation for both Natasha and me that we're not mad, or if we are, we're in very good company.

This is the energy of conception and is happening – whether you are as aware of it as Natasha and Adrian were, or not. It certainly wasn't my experience, more of a 'do we really have to have sex again' after a full week of 'trying'! However you are 'baby dancing' – a lovely term one client describes the lovemaking when trying to conceive – or receiving your baby, you are in the vortex of creation.

I am in awe of Natasha's capacity for love, even throughout all of her most challenging moments. Her kindness and compassion come so naturally. Her willingness to look within and be curious about life, about her 'why', has brought about huge transformations in her life.

Even when we feel we are stuck, when life has thrown huge

curveballs, all is possible. They do not define us. Life changes if we allow it to.

I wish for all of your journeys to unfold and flow as they are meant. As you choose.

# Chapter 6
## Visiting the Spirit Baby Realm.
## A journey into life before life

The following description is how I was shown the spirit baby realm. Maybe others would have different experiences depending on where they're from in the world, but one thing I've come to know from spirit is that they make it relevant to the person they are guiding.

I often wondered what this realm would look like, and often saw it simply as space and stars within which was a transparent dome of life with spirit babies floating around – that was all my limited mind showed me.

I hadn't expected or intended or even thought about asking to be shown the spirit baby realm. It was when I settled down to connect with Rosa, to ask her how and why souls choose their parents, that she invited me to join her there, rather than write her words as I usually do.

Rosa said, "This [earth] is the greatest show to be a part of. With all sorts of gifts and skills they are bringing from all cultures and experiences, here [spirit baby realm] they hone their gifts, make their friends and they plan their lives. Come and see."

I felt nervous. Was this really happening? Was I really going to visit the spirit baby realm? I took a deep breath and went with it. I was sitting in the back of one of my favourite cafés at Merton Abbey Mills in London,  a little oasis of calm near my house where the River Merton runs through – more a stream than a river at this point in its journey. I was the only one in this part of the café that day and so, with the sun streaming through the window, and with a sense of anticipation, I took a breath, smiled and felt myself go into a trance-like state as Rosa lifted me, my consciousness, up and out of my body and I went with wherever I was to be taken.

When Rosa guided me up and up through the limitations of my

mind, my café surroundings and all sense of time melted away. I was there, I was really there. I was given permission to be an observer. My landing point was into what looked and felt like a town, not a UK town, but definitely a town I would recognise as being in the West, not ancient, not modern, it felt dateless.

I watched so many souls walking through the streets, in adult human form, albeit a bit hazy around the edges, as if trying on the form they would take, had already been, or were at least trying on for size. A friendly, happy town. I saw doctors and nurses, carpenters and painters, already practising their future skills and performances. I watched them getting to know, or maybe reacquainting with, their spirit animals who were there to keep them safe and guide them. It was a busy place but tranquil: no rushing, no stress. No sense of aloneness that one can feel among a crowd.

Rosa and I then moved further and further along the long street until we were out of the town and in another place: a space of green hills, sunshine, and a wide blue sky. I felt I was on top of the world. I was told we were in the realm of children who had passed and who wished to come to earth again. It was a beautiful resting place for them to heal and recuperate as they played and waited until they felt the call to take their steps onwards.

The air was fresh and I could hear the laughter of children and could see them playing with dogs and various pets. Animals were quite a prominent feature here and it really struck home to me that spirit animals and our pets here on earth play such a hugely important role in our connection, healing and, of course, the lightness and joy they bring through unconditional love and play.

I saw so many children, again in hazy form, some with a clearer outline than others, playing with hoops – that old-fashioned game of keeping the hoop going whilst running, chasing with such an energy of freedom.

Enjoying the feeling of safety and being back here and free to play for a while, they weren't quite ready to manage the density of the earth world just yet and were simply enjoying themselves without a care in the universe.

As I observed Rosa, or her energy without any form I could recognise, moving onwards, I noticed a band of little souls follow her forward, the ones who were ready to begin their journey back to earth. I joined them as they followed Rosa into what my mind understood to be a school, ready to begin their schooling and their planning for their future lives on earth.

## Location, location, location

In this 'classroom' they could look at the whole earth, an image of the view astronauts are privileged to see, and yet this three-dimensional view could be turned and zoomed in on so they could really get a sense in great detail of all the areas they could go to. Earth under a microscope.

I saw Mount Everest, and as they saw Mount Everest, they all let out a gasp of delight. For many, this felt like a touchstone between earth and this spirit baby realm. An access point perhaps? But the top of Mount Everest was feeling very similar in energy to where they were currently – a precious, spirit-earth connection point. I want to say touching God – or whatever word you prefer to describe that energy of simple stillness and being, that moment we are blessed with every now and again when time seems to stand still. That is what they, and I, felt as this globe honed in on this incredible mountain, as if to reassure them that when they are on earth, they are still connected to heaven.

The children were shown places like Syria and the Middle East and other areas where suffering is a stark reality for so many. They saw what it was like living in the more impoverished places of Africa, but they liked the sense of freedom that being in certain cultures in Africa offers – Africa felt more like 'home'. They were also shown the food eaten by different cultures, including hamburgers in America. Apologies to any Americans reading this, it's not just America that likes hamburgers and I'm partial to one myself occasionally, but to be honest, they did have a giggle at some of the food people were eating!

They were shown the oceans, lakes and seas, the cities and the countryside, the deserts and the forests. And then, finally, the people walking around. I saw a couple walking by an ocean hand in hand, perhaps the future parents of one of these souls.

Where there was less 'light' on the earth to be seen, some of the children became more solemn as they wondered if that was where their light needed to be. Were they drawn to these parts of the world? They knew this would be harder but felt drawn to those places. Some were remembering their own experiences of war.

Syria and the surrounding regions appeared to be a key area of interest for many, and I was told that many of the children in this group had only recently come from there. I watched them watching their parents and families and wondering whether they would see them again, asking if it was their path to go back now with the lessons learnt by the parents and people for whom they had 'sacrificed' their life on earth. Had their passing made a difference to the world then? Would it make a difference now if they came back?

I have to admit I found this aspect pretty distressing. As for all the love, safety, and freedom I had felt in the green hills area among these children, for those whose passing had been more recent and who wanted to return more quickly, there was still deep sadness at what they had experienced and what they were seeing their families going through now.

Some of them felt stronger about going back in, more confident that things had changed and would change again, that they could bring about change. They felt they could make their parents happy again and could see their brothers and sisters and wanted to come back down to comfort them, to help them realise they were still there and hadn't gone.

They could see pockets of light almost like gaps that they could fill.

What was really clear from my almost three-hour journey up into this realm was that location was very important as part of their plan and their mission. Where was their light needed? For example, for some spirits, being by the sea was key. They could see the plastic and knew what they could do to help ease this and so needed to be brought up living by and learning about the sea and marine life. They wanted to play with the whales and the dolphins.

Others, looking at the earth and the pollution, were more drawn to city life as they needed to experience that in order to remind themselves why they were there on earth and what they could do about helping to cleanse and grow the earth. They saw the woods and the fun you can have in nature and wished to show you how you can live with nature once again.

What if your spirit baby was looking down on your life on earth – what would they see? They are looking without judgement; they are looking at location in terms of what they want to do in order to bring light to that particular place.

Basically, they, and I assume that means all of us before we came to earth, were able to view planet Earth from this very high perspective. If we all had the opportunity to be in that space and see our planet and our own lives from this perspective, I wonder if we would do more ourselves to transform how we live and how we treat the earth rather than leaving it all up to this next generation of souls?

## Graduation

And so we moved on to the next stage of the journey back to earth and I was shown a tall red-brick building, like a university. It was obviously a way of representing this stage of graduation in a form I could understand. It was here where all the planners and the masters and the architects of life are to be found – where the more in-depth choices were being made.

I watched the 'grace angels/workers' touch the crown of the souls – touched on the crown by God is what it felt like – and through the door they went with their books and plans in hand, forever and always connected to God and their plan, as they dived into the earth realm.

It was here at this university-type place, that they met up with their soul family members, their friends for life, and began wondering and discussing what each would do. Old loves reunited and agreed to meet up here on earth and where and how, with such a sense of love. They knew they would meet again on earth and have a love interest.

A conversation I heard was:

"Are you coming back?"

"Yes, I'm coming back."

"Where are you going?"

"Okay, I might look into that."

"If you're born there, I'll be born there and we'll arrange to meet here."

There were lots of negotiations and friendships made and reformed, the who, the why, the what, and the where, until all souls found each other to make their plan together.

I got a sense from this particular snapshot that, on the whole, location was a key choice as part of their why. The next choice was who they were to be with in this life and, finally, how they were to be born. I'm aware this sounds quite simplistic and I know that planning is much bigger than any of us can imagine. There's always a bigger, bigger plan. But I believe what I was shown is a snapshot of how an individual plan comes together – our own piece of an infinite puzzle.

## How do souls choose their parents?

Some parents are already chosen from the soul family and they go first into the world, of course. I saw a dad-type figure saying, "Goodbye and see you soon," to a son-type energy figure. There was role-swapping being arranged, with souls who had played the role of mum becoming a friend, or children becoming the parent, all swapping roles and making negotiations and agreements. And others choosing soul family members whom they knew would offer them the experiences they needed.

Some souls hadn't chosen parents first and began to look for them in the location they had chosen; people they thought looked nice in the location that they wanted. I also heard souls asking to 'meet up with' soul family members who had recently passed as they knew they could offer them insight, wisdom, and advice before they arrived on earth.

Others looked into potential parents and some had a few options they couldn't decide between, as all would offer the love they needed and they wanted to spend time with each one.

Souls already here on earth would then come to their own place of knowing about having a baby, and soul contracts, if not negotiated previously, would happen between the higher selves, although I wasn't shown how this takes place. I also understand that these agreements are continuously updated throughout conception, birth and beyond.

They didn't see anyone we here on earth may feel or deem to be a 'bad' choice because these souls weren't judging the behaviour of anyone. They only saw the love and the light of the souls.

I spent time with one beautiful soul and they were observing their future parents in a dingy and dirty tiny kitchen, a couple not looking after themselves too well – at least from my own point of judgement at the time. I'm sure we all have that question as to why children would choose what may be considered by many as a challenging family upbringing.

"Because I love them," they stated simply. "I want to be with them because I love them and they can give me what I need and bring me to where I need to go and because I'll be different, I can help them to be different too."

I saw many guides talking to the baby souls and, although my knowledge of sacred geometry is minimal, there were symbols, diagrams and charts, maps of the stars that showed how everything is aligning and how we'll all align in this huge picture of the universe. I can only describe it as how I imagine a strategy room looks in those old World War Two films, with maps and figures being manoeuvred about but on a massive scale.

Not all of the souls I saw at this 'university' went to the next stage of their earth birth. Some chose to stay behind and advise here about their time on earth and share their stories and information.

Some simply changed their minds and left the university for a while to go elsewhere at that time. And some returned to the green hills area for more healing and play, not yet ready or because it was not their time.

I know for sure I was only shown a tiny glimpse of what goes on in the preparations for coming to earth. As a Soul Plan Reader I can access an individual's 'planning room', their immediate life before life, so they can gain a personal perspective of their choices in this lifetime, why their life is as it is, what they came in with – their why and their what. And if you choose to, you can gain a fuller picture of who you truly are, the aspects of yourself from the very beginning of time. It is quite profound when you acknowledge the hugeness of yourself and all that you've been and experienced. Without meaning to sound flippant, in comparison, this lifetime should be a doddle!

It was quite some journey up into this realm, almost three hours in which I hadn't noticed anything else going on in the café, and I got a parking ticket for going over time. Well, it was an expensive cup of coffee but oh so worth it and I hope it helps in some way with either the joy of knowing your baby who chose not to stay is totally happy playing in the green hills, or that your future baby is looking over you, waiting for their time and your time to be right to come together on earth. Your little piece of heaven coming to you.

Rosa also confirmed to me that she and I had met here before. That she is one of the teachers and advisors in the 'University'. "It was my choice to come to you in form so we could reconnect you with me, with us, with here," she said. Incidentally, I also saw my best friend Sam there.

# Chapter 7
# The Many Ways of Coming into the World.
## IVF and egg donation

I mentioned in the soul's checklist of planning that one of the choices souls make is how they wish to arrive and how they wish their birth experience to be. Knowing that they too are involved in this choice, it's helpful to stay open to how your little ones arrive in your life, which can help take the pressure off in terms of how you think it 'should' happen.

IVF may be a medical process, however, the spark of life, the spark of creation, is very far from the control of medical science.

I personally believe, and there is much evidence and babies in the world which demonstrate this belief, that IVF is not always a necessary route to go down if there is no medical, physical reason why pregnancy doesn't happen.

As you will read throughout this book, conception isn't just a physical act. It is a journey that you, your baby (and partner, if you have one) are on. You will read in the coming chapters the many beliefs and traumas, known and unknown, that may be affecting the way your body reacts to these often hidden thoughts that are preventing conception. There is, of course, also your timing, your babies being ready, and divine timing.

The IVF process itself is extremely wearing and challenging physically and emotionally, creating huge stress. Not to mention the trauma of your journey in coming to this choice in the first place. If you are reading this and are thinking about IVF, or have been through an unsuccessful IVF process, then I hope these insights and Rosa's words hold you in love and allow you to see your journey from a different perspective.

We can spend years and thousands of pounds trying to get pregnant through medical intervention – feeling ever more angry, upset, shut down, and that life is simply not fair. And so perhaps this book will be the start of your inner journey to understand why it is and what may be holding you back – and yes, even why your baby is holding back on arriving.

Please know they are not holding back because there's something 'wrong' with you. They love you unconditionally; you are already perfect. They have chosen you. They view their holding back as offering a gift to you – the gift of healing. They want you to see yourself through their eyes and not in terms of the negative thought patterns you may have about yourself – which are simply untrue. I hope that you'll begin to look within a little more, without judgement. Be very, very kind to yourself.

When IVF is the chosen route – by you and your future baby or babies – it's so important to find healing, peace, and resolution in regard to any previous attempts. If you have experienced one or more unsuccessful IVF treatment, imagine the fear, trauma, stress, and mistrust held in your body from this. I totally understand how infuriating it is when someone says to you 'just relax and it will happen'. Whether we're trying to get pregnant or not there's no question, however, that finding ways to relax our mind and body boosts our health and balances our hormones. The more we can find balance the less we're pumping out the stress hormones of adrenaline and cortisol that inhibit a clear mind, our digestive system, and reproductive system.

Without adding even more pressure on yourself of being 'perfect', or I must do this, or kicking yourself by believing it's not working because I had a glass of wine, for example, please remember you are already perfect. Do not buy into the belief you're not pregnant yet because it's all your fault. So many women come to me feeling like a failure, and it's no surprise when they've heard the language of 'failed cycle', or 'failed to embed'. There is so much more going on and it's not all down to you. You're not, and it's not, a failure: your baby has a choice in when, where, and how just as much as you do.

For your own emotional and mental wellbeing, be curious if there are ways of bringing more calm into your day. Even three deep breaths before you leave the house make all the difference. Going into the IVF process feeling emotionally strong, supported, confident, trusting, and open to the process will make your entire experience go with much more ease and flow emotionally.

If you're asking how this might be possible – it begins with self-awareness and your mindset. IVF and other medical processes are very much focused on the physical aspect and I despair when a woman's mental and emotional health isn't supported alongside this. Take a look into counselling and/or energy healing practices such as Reiki, EFT, Matrix Birth Reimprinting, Theta Healing, Spiritual Healing, IET, or reflexology – there are an abundance of tools and gifted practitioners out there who can guide you. You'll be guided to the therapy and the practitioner that you are meant to find.

We are energy – emotions are e-motion, energy in motion – and for life to flow we need to allow our emotions to flow; although so often it seems easier to ignore them, bury them, be stuck in them. By exploring our emotions, we realise they are merely our signposts to what is truly going on underneath the layers of life.

This will be covered more in the following chapter looking at transforming your beliefs, finding resolution and a deep understanding of any trauma, learning to trust and reducing stress. For now, here are some spiritual insights into the reasons why babies may wish to arrive through IVF, egg donation, or adoption.

## Why do babies choose to arrive through IVF?

### According to Rosa:

Your babies have a choice in all things and they may not choose IVF, but they do choose you. And so, if IVF or any other medical procedure is what is happening, then it makes no matter to them in which way they arrive. Their only thought is that they do arrive with you at some point in time, whether in this lifetime or the next, for there is always a connection between you as a soul and the baby as a soul who is ready to be rebirthed in the world. It is simply a matter of the when.

And that is more complex than what you can see. But what I wish you to know is: the choice of your baby is their choice of you. They choose you. How does that make you feel if you are going through a difficult procedure? Your babies choose you. What would you do differently, or rather, how differently would you feel going into these processes knowing this?

What would you feel if you know that they have chosen you and are simply waiting for you to be ready for them, whether emotionally or physically? They know when they are ready and they also know when you are ready to receive them. So what is it that needs to happen within you, within your mind and your psyche, to allow yourself to receive them?

Is it fear? Is it desperation? Is it powerlessness or mistrust? What is it that you need from your baby? What is it that your journey is showing you about yourself, about your wounds and your joy – and how is it that the joy in you, the love in you, can outwit and ease this energy of fear, self-doubt and of punishment and persecution?

It is something I would like you to think about, to feel about, as you go on your journey to motherhood – no matter which way this is coming for you. It is you, it is always you, who holds the key and the answers. It is in spite of and not because of the science of IVF.

In this, women should take heart in their own power and their ability to create, because it was not the IVF that brought their baby to them, but they who brought and can bring their baby to them.

This may not make sense to those who have welcomed their baby through IVF, for of course they are grateful for the science that allowed this physical act to come to fruition. But please read my words carefully, feel them deeply:

*'it is in spite of the IVF process, and not because of it, that your baby soul came to you'.*

You must know that your power to create birthed your baby

into life and not the power of the medical procedure. So please take heart, all of you women who are going down this route of IVF, for those of you who have yet to meet them in physical form – it is you – it is always you who holds the power to create, to hold the life-force energy of another, and to grow and nurture that life form into the physical home, the body of your baby soul.

It is not the physical, it is you. And so, if you are entering into this process in order to meet your baby, do so with an open mind as to your own power, your own right to create, for that is what you are here for – to create life – your life, as well as the life of another, if that is part of your soul's wishes.

So do not hand over your power to the science and the medical, be in the power of you as you utilise the inspiration and the genius of the science and the medical, but always be in no doubt that it is you who is the creator.

And so it is.

As with everything there is always, always a much bigger picture to what we are seeing and experiencing. There is more discussion on the energy behind the need and inspiration for IVF in Part 3 of this book, which looks at the collective.

## Why do some babies choose to arrive through egg donation?

For many, this is the final option in terms of carrying a child. There can be a sense of uneasiness around egg donation largely because of the question: is the baby really mine? And I truly hope the message below, which comes through Lady Venus rather than Rosa, tips this on its head and into a new perspective. I'm not sure why Lady Venus came in to deliver this message but I'm sure we'll find the answer one day.

It is I (Lady Venus) who can talk to you about egg donation, my dear. For when is a soul not a soul? When is a soul ever what a soul is, and when is a soul ever what a soul is not?

Do you see, a soul is a soul no matter the form or the body it comes in? Do you see, sometimes a soul wishes to come in to a particular form? Often this form is not able to be provided by its chosen parents. Therefore the soul then has a choice – re-choose its parents, or choose again the body it would like to experience within its chosen parents.

Do you see, that it makes no matter, what matter (body) the soul arrives in, from its perspective? For what it is choosing as a soul is to experience life with a particular physicality and a physicality that may not be able to be physically provided by its parents.

And so, either its parents have to change or the path is set for the right egg and the right physicality to be placed within the parents.

It is not a curse at all that some of your women are having to go down this route of what can be seen as a last resort, when in fact the baby soul is so keen, so set and so in love with its chosen parents, that it is prepared to move with the machinations of the universe in order to not only remain with this choice of parents, because of a love so strong nothing will change their minds about it, but also because of their wish to experience whatever is in the genes and the make-up of the body that they desire.

We know that this is not an easy choice for the women and indeed not even the men for there is a certain sense of ownership that comes when we become pregnant with our baby child. We may find it difficult to let go of that ownership, that sense that something is yours and yours alone and you made and created it and you have this baby soul all to yourself as yours and no one else's.

Perhaps the agreement between this baby soul and its

parents is exactly to help the parents with this sense of ownership and learn this lesson, albeit a difficult one. That you cannot own a soul and you cannot own a life and you cannot make or create a soul for the soul is already whole.

As you become a parent, that which you are doing is merely birthing this soul into this life. You cannot own it, for it is not to be owned, it can only be owned by itself and for itself. In that ownership, it has chosen for you to be the vessel, the creator, the womb, of the physical body, whether that is the physical body of your own physical body, or not.

So please take heart, our beautiful women of light, who here come across this particular soul's choice. Know that you are indeed of the highest vibration if you are able to take on and accept this concept of a free-flowing universe in which nothing and no one can be owned, and that even if this soul is not of your own physical body, it is your soul they have chosen to be birthed in, by and to.

The love these baby souls have for you knows no bounds. They are limitless in their choices and yet they have chosen you. They have chosen you because of the love they have for you. They have chosen you because of the history they have with you. They have chosen you because you are you. And they wish for you to love you, just as they love you. With no ownership of mind, body, or soul, only a simple knowing that it is you who are to be together again in this lifetime.

And so it is.

I was also asked to look at the experience of egg donation from the perspective of the donor. This question sparked the most massive download of information about eggs, sperm, creation, choice, and the true limitless beings we are. It blew my mind a bit and I'm still working through the message myself!

Our human minds can find it hard to process intangibles so stay open to all that you read from Rosa, you'll take in what you're ready for and each time you grow into yourself and your understanding, you'll take on board more and more depth. This is the beauty of being curious.

I sat down to hear Rosa's words and instead was taken on a surprise journey into the 'entrance' of the Universe. In my mind it was a vulva of light and the journey through this portal into the entrance of life was the most incredible feeling of joy and love.

I did my usual 'I haven't got much time to go on any journeys today, please can I just have the message!' and was told by Rosa to always look for another way and perspective, so I surrendered into it. I let go into deep meditation and, as always, I'm so glad I did because the images I was shown, like watching a movie, helped me to make so much more sense of the words that followed.

Through this entrance, this portal, I was shown the image of a giant egg. It looked a little flimsy around the edges and weak in its energy, fragile, and even felt a little damaged. I was told that sperm would be able to access this egg easily because it is weakened energetically, however, it is not a life force energy that will be strong enough to turn into an embryo.

I was then shown another egg that seemed to be glowing, pulsing with light, with much stronger boundaries and feeling very 'upright'. If this egg was a woman she'd be standing tall holding her head high.

## Rosa on eggs, sperm, creation, and choice

The energy of the egg is weakened by the constant abuse of the woman. Whether this is by their own thoughts that they are defective or whether it is a lifelong battle to feel strong in themselves, a person in their own right; an energy that has boundaries and knows to stand in their own power. A woman who is loved equals an egg who is loved.

The egg is also weakened by the life of the woman's mother. Did the mother wish to become pregnant? What does the mother think of her child? Did the woman, as a girl, feel wanted or not wanted? If she didn't feel wanted is it then wrong to want a child of her own?

All of this affects the egg because it is an energy that affects you, the woman. So what is carried in the person is carried in the egg.

There are no limits to the coding that is held in an egg and so the information held in the egg can be limitless. It is the coding of the sperm and the beliefs of the sperm and the DNA of the sperm that will mix and match – to match the exact same frequency as demanded by the child who is to fill the embryo.

Do you see that it is the egg and the sperm that hold infinite possibility and infinite timelines, and the child, the soul who is able to decode the code to the one they wish to carry as a mix of the two experiences, that is the crux of the issue here.

So they will pick out the code of memories they wish to have, the traumas they wish to feel, the junk they wish to get rid of – the infinite possibility that is the sperm and the egg.

So the egg of a donor and the sperm of a donor do not make matter (form) of what matters. It is the energy of the egg and the energy of the sperm that does make the matter (body) because the baby child knows exactly which of the coding from within both the egg and the sperm that it wishes to experience.

So for those who receive the donor egg and donor sperm, it is for their baby to make the choice as to which egg and sperm, within the infinite possibility they contain, and also within the parameters of what's possible for the human mum and dad to access and align with. (Accept and hold in their body and lives)

We are told to do so much to improve the physical quality of our eggs, through diet, exercise, and self-care, and Rosa's message also shows how important it is to look at your family history, your experience as an egg in the womb of your mum, your mum's experience of conception and birth as well as your own. It all sounds so complicated but please be reassured it's not. Your emotions and thoughts are signposts to any healing that may need to happen to help you feel stronger, more you and less the layers of life that feel heavy. This in turn has an effect on your eggs.

If nothing else, this message confirms that your babies have choice, right from the outset. And as you were once in the spirit baby realm contemplating arriving here on earth, gain strength from knowing that you too made these choices, had choice, right at the very beginning. You still have choice. Choose you.

One consistent message from the spirit babies is: find you, find us. Your journey to motherhood can be one big kick up the bum to bring you onto the path of finding yourself, your true self; not what you've been told you are or should be by others. The babies of the New Earth have lived many lives and choices and wish to arrive more 'awake' now than ever before. In order for them to have greater choice, healing yourself, healing your eggs (and sperm) offers this. You are lifting your energy, your vibration, to be a more equal match to their very high vibration.

**A message to donors from Rosa**

> It is the donors of these 'codes' we must now turn. Because there are some who will wish to spread their code with light and some who wish to spread with dark. So the parents of the future child must be careful to pick the exact energy they wish for the experience they wish for themselves and their children. And they may not know what this is on a conscious level – but they will 'know' what are the right egg and sperm donor for what is meant to be. (Intuition)
>
> And so the darker donors – all I mean by this is that they are not giving with love and from love. So for many of them, their eggs will be null and void at any cost because it is ultimately

the baby spirit who will choose the egg and the sperm that is matched with their intention and then again the choose the exact coding available within this egg and sperm that they wish to experience.

Parents be reassured that the margin of error is very much at a minimum at any time in the best of ways because there is always a choice.

Some baby souls may wish to experience the lack of love in which they were given and that is a fine thing because it is a lesson and a choice they wish to experience. So do you see when it comes to donors there must always be a choice too of whether to give in love or whether to give in desperation or give in fear.

And this is okay because some baby souls may choose to feel this. However many now will not – and so therefore the experimentation that is necessary in order to extract an egg makes this pretty much null and void. Therefore is there any point in giving in desperation and giving into the hope when it is unlikely that this will result in a live birth?

So what we would say to all donors who are going down the line of giving,  is to ask: why you are giving? Are you giving for your own selfish reasons of fear of money, of lack, of not being able to produce a live baby of your own, or are you giving from love? Love of another and love of the future baby soul who will be picking the coding from your infinite source of energy that is contained in that sample of sperm or contained in the whole of the egg?

And what is it that this giving is making you feel? Because just as the baby souls are choosing their experience, so too are you. So what is it you are choosing to experience, in this experience? Is it love? Is it denial? Is it faith in humanity? Is it fear of being given away yourself that is driving the fear of you having to give away something of yourself?

This message could go on and on as the infinite possibility

because this is what happens here, infinite possibilities. What you need to know in its simplest terms is that the energy you put into your giving is the exact same energy that you put into your receiving.

So, if you do not choose to give of yourself in your current state of un-love, then you will not receive the energy of un-love back. Do you see your energy of un-loved may well come back to you in infinite ways because you have helped create this energy of un-love in another soul? This is not a bad thing because some souls may well likely have wished to experience the energy of un-love itself – and so you were matched.

But it also means this cycle of un-love continues. And this cannot be the way of the world any longer, for these new souls will not accept the energy of un-love – they will only accept the energy of all love. The love that is the beauty of creation and duplication of the All that is love.

So if you do not wish to continue to feel the energy of un-love – then do not give this energy out any longer in any form. And if you still wish to give but from a place of love, then it is time for your own coding to be released and transformed from one of un-love to love. From one of trauma and abandonment, or one of not-enoughness, into the whole and light soul you are at heart.

Do you see that just as the journey to motherhood, parenthood, is the soul's journey, so is the journey to giving by the donor part of their own soul's growth. So we would encourage any soul who is thinking of donating to think again of the energy they are putting out into the world and the energy they wish to receive back.

Because this is the truth of the matter, that it is the truth that creates matter (form/body).

And so it is.

The first time I read this message back I noticed I felt some fear around it. Egg donation wasn't my path but I know the questions and fears my clients go through when making this choice. I had to step back for a while, re-read the message and look at which parts of it created fear. For me, it was the thought of coming from an unloved egg and sperm, being unloved. Also, my eggs being unloved and therefore passing this onto my children and out into the world – yikes, that's a huge responsibility and the next thought was: how rubbish am I! There are signposts to healing in everything and I was able to release this belief as it's not something I wish to be carrying or projecting. We'll look at how you can transform beliefs in the chapters further on.

You'll have noticed different emotions reading this message. Breathe, nothing is wrong, you haven't done or not done anything wrong or made a wrong choice. Remember your baby has the choice as to what they wish to take on and experience. They have their own journey. If it is un-love, as Rosa refers to a lack of love, this is their choice and through your own healing, you'll be better able to empower and guide them to remember the love they are. It's a journey. What Rosa is saying is that the baby souls now arriving are more often choosing to feel love from the outset. You have a choice in this.

Above all else, remember her words – there is very little margin for error. Whether you are strongly intuitively called to a particular donor and have a knowing, or not, behind the scenes there is so much going on to bring you, your donor, and your baby together. The picture is huge! Trusting yourself and your baby is key.

I have to admit I don't know much about how fertility clinics choose their donors and the background checks they make, but wouldn't it be great if each donor received counselling and healing too before they went ahead.

There's always healing to be done and so feeling these emotions and thoughts is so important. Don't shy away from them, be curious as to why they are there, they are your access point to clearing out the junk you don't need and discovering the light and truth of you underneath it. Don't make it mean anything about you other than a joy at discovering another area you can let go of.

An egg that feels strong, loved, is the reflection of the woman who carries her. As it is for the man. Slowly, slowly, this is how we build a New Earth, knowing all the while, everything is perfect.

Your babies have many ingenious ways of coming together with you for many unique reasons. Adoption is another way we come together. I have written a section on adoption in Part 3 of the book because the message offers insight into the bigger, bigger universal picture going on.

# Birth choices

It's not only conception or how you find each other that there is a choice around. A whole other book could cover why you and your babies may choose a particular type of birth experience. If you wish to look into this more, I highly recommend Sharon King's Heal Your Birth, Heal Your Life. She is the creator of Birth Matrix Reimprinting, a protocol which guides you to rewrite your birth experience. I also recommend a wonderful book (that is pretty hard to get a hold of) called Being Born by Robyn Furnance.

From my own experience as a Soul Plan Reader, I've noticed a correlation between the type of birth experience, and the traits and beliefs that come with this experience, which seem to activate challenges in our soul plan that we need to understand and resolve. My eldest son Max's birth was pretty traumatic for many reasons. In terms of this aspect, however, the experience was that he became stuck and needed assistance to come out using a ventouse.

The traits of this type of birth are feelings of dependency, needing help, feeling like they can't do things alone. These are very similar to the energy of Max's soul's choice of worldly challenge and associated beliefs, such as: I am a failure, I need help, I'm not ready, and I'll mess up.

How this challenge played out for Max in his early years was wanting to do something like joining in at a party, but holding himself back. He was very dependent on either me or my husband being with him. I have since gone back to Max's birth many times and transformed how both he and I felt about it through Matrix Birth Reimprinting. Since then, from age five, all of this changed for him. Max is a beautiful soul, wise beyond his years, very aware and empathic. He's continually growing in his independence, and most definitely I and my husband noticed a huge change in him after easing the trauma around his birth.

My youngest son's birth was beautiful right up until the end when the midwife noticed the cord was wrapped around his neck. The trait that souls wish to experience around this type of birth is basically to be a daredevil, to take risks. Oh yes, this is him! His soul's choice of challenge is all about power and working through what power means. Is it having power over or giving away power? We all work through our sense of what it means to be in our power.

Essentially power is having a stable and strong sense of self-belief, having nothing to prove. The greatest leaders are those who, through their own sense of self-worth, encourage and guide others to be their own leaders.

For Samuel and his soul plan challenge, the associated beliefs include: I need drama to feel alive and I need to cause trouble to get noticed. Samuel is an incredible character with so much joy and life in him. He has the most generous and loving heart with powerful, high vibration healing energies in his chart. Being aware of both of our boys' soul challenges and their gifts, my husband, Lee, and I are better able to guide them on their own path to embrace all of who they are. Fun and games it will be!

It's worth taking a moment to think about your own birth experience. What do you consciously know about your birth? It is incredible the beliefs and decisions you can make about yourself and the world at birth, many of which are so deeply ingrained they colour all aspects of your life. They can also affect your journey to motherhood. If your own birth didn't feel safe for physical or emotional reasons, for example, this can lead to fears around giving birth, which can, in turn, subconsciously affect your health with conditions such as endometriosis, and also affect you becoming pregnant. A sense of lack of love, separation, conflict or trauma going back along your female line impacts how you see and live life, affects your own birth and the birth of your children. Bonding and breastfeeding issues, and post-natal depression, can signify where deeper healing is required.

One of my clients, now a friend, is an intuitive, trauma-informed midwife, breastfeeding counsellor and powerful fellow healer who supports women through pregnancy and birth. Alison Shaloe communicates with babies in the womb and at birth as they share their needs with her and what's going on for them. Just incredible. Her channelled writing below of her own baby self in the womb may help to explain how a baby feels in the womb, the decisions they make, and how you as a conscious and aware mum can help give yourself and your baby the most beautiful, nourishing pregnancy and birth experience.

**Alison's message in poem form from her baby self in the womb:**

When I was just a baby

Not even fully grown

I was in my mother's womb

But wasn't in there alone

I was surrounded by love

But also anxiety and fear

You see she lost her baby

Her son she held most dear

Her pain was my pain

That I cannot deny

She was bereft and sad

Her emotions did not lie

I felt her deepest grief
So saddened by her loss
It was that time that I agreed
To help her and be Boss

I promised to take care of her
And support her all her life
I did this with much pride
Even though there was struggle and strife
No one would have noticed
But I carried her pain in me
Her emotional ups and downs
Were silently present in me
I came to this world
With a knowing in my heart
That no matter what we went through
We would never be apart
Her love for me is never-ending
I knew it from the start
There was this inner knowing
That this love was from her heart

Women have been wounded
For as long as we know
So now the time has come
For women to start to grow
It's time to address
The underlying hurt

The guilt and shame
Hidden beneath the dirt
We live in a patriarchy
Over-ruled by men
And now it's time for the matriarchy
To start to rule again
Women are creative
They have their wombs for this
We just need to clear the space
To make it hers, not his!

For she is very strong
And a threat to humankind
So that is why these men
Have tried to make her blind
For we have seen the truth
Of who we really are
We just need the courage
To stand up and raise the bar
For too long we've been silenced
But not so any more
Dealing with the traumas
That are really at the core
We are not our stories
We are not our past
We are so much more than that
Our world is changing fast

Such a beautiful poem that highlights the soul journey from conception.

Our bodies are affected by our environment, including the environment of our minds. Finding out what is lurking there is essential to our health and well-being and what we are creating in our life.

# Chapter 8
# Creating Life
# Why do some babies wait so long to arrive?

What do baby souls want? How can the waiting for your spirit babies, or the loss of them, be a gift?

Now you are aware of the journey you are on together with your baby, and the choices they make, the next question is: why do they choose not to arrive or choose not to stay?

The consistent message from Rosa, from Source, from the baby spirits themselves, is that the souls who are ready, and have chosen to be birthed on earth, are choosing and asking their parents and their parents-to-be, to become more self-aware, to heal their traumas and shed their layers in order to allow in more of the lighter energies.

By doing so, these parents not only start to feel more whole, more themselves for their own benefit, energetically they are clearing space, emptying themselves of the lower vibration energies such as guilt and resentment, to hold the light of their babies. They will also be able to better guide and support these beautiful souls in their own mission once they arrive.

We have already been shown that the new baby souls waiting to arrive are of a higher vibration. The following message from Rosa offers us an insight into these souls and their journey from the baby spirit world to here.

So whether you have a child, are pregnant, have lost a baby, or are waiting for one, I hope that Rosa's message will bring you some comfort and the insight that your babies really do have their own journeys and choices and that their love for you is limitless and beyond the physical.

## Rosa's message on the journey from spirit realm to earth realm

And so, my little one, let us begin with the art of loss, for loss is an art to be practised and experienced and journeyed through.

Our babies can offer us this opportunity to experience loss and journey through the darkness that it brings in order to bring us to the other side of the light and the knowing and the feeling that your babies are indeed still with you, and therefore you have learnt and understood the beautiful lesson that no one ever truly dies and you are always connected to them and to the light.

For the baby spirits that are coming through to you now are the ones that are of the light, and the ones who are also closest to the earth and closest to their transition time, as they move and shift their own vibrations to a deeper resonance of the world you live in in order to prepare for this transition.

Maybe you would like to know how this transition occurs? This may perhaps alleviate some of the questions and concerns of all your mums-to-be, and of all grandmothers, sisters and friends of these mums, who too are waiting to take up their role as guardians of the little souls. Souls who show their bravery and courage in coming into the world at this time in order to heal the world of all the past angsts, wars and worries that have been experienced there.

For these little souls are truly brave and special and have a much higher light, and therefore it takes them that bit longer to dull their light, if you like, in order to weigh themselves down and become used to the ways of the world and the density they can so often feel there.

They often need to practice this density feeling and that may mean popping in and out of their chosen bodies until they can adjust and feel comfortable with the physical weight of a body.

Then they must also find or wait for their chosen parents to also lift their vibration in order that they are a vibrational match on this planet as well as in spirit.

So do you see how important it is for your mums, and also your dads, to be prepared for this shift in energy too? That they feel able to hold this amount of light in their bodies and in their life. So they must turn to making space in their bodies by releasing all that no longer serves them and closing off the space between the energy of their babies and the energy in this world.

Once our babies of light here have practised for some time living and not living in the density of your world, there comes a time when they are ready to move and shift their vibration in such a way that their body becomes a form in which they are comfortable being housed for the duration of their life on this planet.

It's truly incredible how we get here.

As Rosa tells us, it may take a while for babies to practise being in the density of the world. Sometimes this is what they are doing when they only stay a short time. They may also have some more preparation work of their own to do before they arrive, or are waiting for the right time, for them, for you, for whatever the timing of the bigger, bigger plan is. You are not alone on this journey. It is also the journey of your babies and future babies.

**Rosa shares her insight**

My darling ladies, it is with great pleasure that I connect with you all to let you know that you are all doing so well and we here are all very proud of you.

We know that this is a difficult journey to undertake and one that has many pitfalls and low moments but we ask that you continue to hold the faith in us for we too are doing our work up here in order to prepare for our arrival into your world, and yes, into your arms.

This is a very special time and a sacred moment that cannot be rushed and we ask you to please be patient for the agreements you have made are sure to come to pass when all is in place for the arrival of these beings who are coming here in order to save the world, save the world from themselves and itself.

So, do not be frightened by this and do not think this is too big a task for you as parents, because it is not. It is indeed the way it was always meant to be and always will be.

They are coming, but they have a very special task to perform and for that they too have to be prepared. Know this at your core and give them the time and space they will need not only as they transition but also as they arrive and begin their lifelong journeys with you.

I know there is patience to be had, however patience is always rewarded with the kindest and most special of souls and of this we can promise.

So, hold yourselves and hold your light in our eyes, in our hearts, in our minds, for they are surely coming to you when the moment is right.

And it is also important to share this message with others, because those of you who are so far without, are those of you who must also go within. For there is a great tide that is turning in your world and you, my darling ones, are the ones who have chosen to lift it and ride it and travel on it until the ends of time in a most glorious way of enlightenment.

As you read earlier, babies who choose not to stay often come in for a brief time to help their parents to awaken to the possibility that there are other realms, that there is more going on behind the scenes than you can physically see, or that your mind can comprehend. That there is life after death and life before life.

The babies wishing to come in are also waiting for their mums and dads to be in a clearer space in mind, body, and spirit.

This is not to pile even more pressure on you, but to invite you to take a different perspective. They are not saying you need to have completely cleared all your traumas and limitations – as we all know this is a lifelong journey – simply to become more self-aware.

What I have discovered working with mums-in-waiting, is that each baby requires their chosen parents to have shifted something unique to their contract, or needs. A common theme has been around power. There is always a much bigger picture going on than what we can see, and the journey to motherhood offers a very clear example of how the imbalance of power between the masculine and the feminine energies shows up. You'll read more on this in Part 2 and 3 when we turn to the collective.

For now, for you, spirit babies want their mums to at the very least recognise their power; to stop giving away the power by going along with someone else's idea of what is right or fun, what they should and should not do, and what is possible or not possible for them. This is the deep wound of the mother, not being 'allowed' or not feeling safe to be themselves, and ultimately a receiver and creator of life. This is why I say women going through challenges to become pregnant are the most courageous, deeply loving souls because on the soul level, on an unconscious level, they wish to remember and reclaim their own sense of self and power. And this can be no easy task. Through the darkness of the womb and into the light of themselves as I've mentioned before.

One beautiful spirit baby, now very much in the world with their equally fabulous twin, was very specific. She wanted their mum to trust herself and her intuition and not simply allow the doctors to take over during her IVF process. She had to practise being in her power. This story becomes even more relevant in Part 3 of this book on the bigger picture. Remember Rosa's earlier message about how it is you, the woman, the creator, who holds the power to bring in and hold the life-force energy of your baby, utilising scientific and medical knowledge if needs be? Jules' story is a clear example of this.

## Julie tells her story

I met my partner when I was around 35 or 36. After a year, we decided to try and get pregnant. It didn't worry me that we weren't married. In the back of my mind, I was wondering about fertility, but to the fore of my mind, everything was great and I felt excited and told loads of friends!

Years went by. We did tests, but nothing showed up, only that I had PCOS (Polycystic Ovary Syndrome) and my AMH (Anti-Müllerian hormone) was dropping as I was getting older. We tried Clomid and timed intercourse – fun times! IVF was suggested and I was starting to panic about my age, so I jumped into IVF treatment in Prague.

We had success – six blastocytes and two transferred, which took. Twins! But at eight weeks we had a miscarriage which, rightly or wrongly, I blamed on the early scan. I knew it hadn't felt right to do the scan but went against my own knowing and followed the medical advice.

We had four more blastocysts frozen so went back twice with no success each time. I felt deflated and older and fed up of the rollercoaster of emotions, choosing the right healthy foods and not drinking to drown my sorrows. I felt very sorry for myself and started to resent others who became pregnant so easily naturally – and for free!

I felt like a failure and that I'd let my partner down. It was all my fault. His friends getting pregnant hit me harder than my own friends' pregnancies. I took time off to try to get pregnant naturally, to stop trying, as people always say when you stop trying it works.

I was thinking: I'm 40 next year. I'm doing everything from supplements to a healthy diet and moderate exercise, alternative therapists, and vision boards. What more could I do? What was I not doing?

On Facebook, I saw that one of my brother's friends was doing kundalini yoga online. I love yoga and didn't know a lot about kundalini, but I was intrigued by the idea of doing my own yoga at home and it seemed more spiritual.

I was excited to challenge myself to do something different just for me. I shared my journey with the teacher, Linda Martin, who told me about Debra. Again, something different, but I took a leap and trusted. I signed up to work with Debra, initially looking at my Soul Plan Reading, which was insightful, to say the least, and very much around my sense of disempowerment that stretched back long before this lifetime. We then had sessions around fertility, going deep into this lifetime and other lifetime traumas, including, of course, understanding and healing the beliefs about myself and my fertility journey and the miscarriages.

After my inner work, I was feeling happier, calmer and more content. Life just seemed to flow easier. I had decided to go to London for IVF. It was a more intense treatment than Prague, and I had to go over and back a lot for all the tests. It was also a lot more money and it took a longer time. But I felt ready.

I had changed to a very good work environment and was now taking each step as it came. I wasn't the type to travel solo but somehow I was flying to London on my own for day trips. I did a workshop with another lady in Ireland and focused on fertility but realised that I had already done the work with Debra. I felt relaxed, like all had been released.

After that, things fell into place. When I was ready to go to London my brother happened to be home, so I flew back with him and I stayed with him for three weeks and then with my other brother for another three weeks. I was independent in London, going to the clinic each day, something I hadn't really been doing before. I also used the time to focus on myself; again usually I would get into other people's stuff and tell everyone my stuff. I reserved my energy for myself and when I needed an ear, I contacted Debra, and she very much gave me spot-on advice, as well as reminding me to ground myself and the clinic and clear the space.

Even the moon cycles seemed to tie in with the timing of the transfer. I'd noticed how I was feeling at each phase of the moon and knew I felt most alive at the full moon. The day of the transfer was a full moon.

I even decided, just before my transfer and after Debra's meditation, where the goddess Brigid came in to assist with healing and messages, that if I had a girl I'd call her Brigid, after my granny and the goddess of fertility – I stuck to that promise! I look back on that IVF journey now with joy. It was an enjoyable, challenging experience, something I didn't feel about my previous IVF cycles. Of course it all going my way helped.

Now as a mum of seven-month-old twins, as I write this, I feel hugely grateful, excited and sometimes still shocked! Debra sent me a painting of an angel with two babies. I looked at it for strength in the early weeks of overwhelm, hormones and no sleep! Having them reminds me of another time of healing, something physical I was going through – it's a miracle! And miracles do happen, as I said to my friend who's doing IVF now, and to all of you who are going through this. I send my love.

Julie's story shows how by going within, being courageous and open to finding you underneath the layers of life, the beliefs and the pain, transforms how you feel about yourself and your life journey. And if it's meant to be, creating your life with your babies here.

I'm not saying this is easy and I know Julie put into practice all the insights and learnings from her babies and her own inner knowing, learning how to say no to others and yes to herself. Among the myriad of emotions that arise on a challenging journey to motherhood, sadness is one of them. It's okay to be sad. It's also good to delve into the sadness a little and what is lying underneath because often this is a feeling of helplessness. Rosa's messages are very direct in saying you are not helpless. You are powerful and you own so many gifts, are the gift that can lift you back into the knowledge of your power and self-belief.

Julie's babies were very forthright when they connected with her, outlining what they wished for her to look at. Other spirit babies have encouraged their mums to put themselves first or to speak out. One baby asked her mum to find her 'Mama Bear' spirit because she was going to need her mum to be fiercely loving and protective. She was a live wire and her mum was going to need to be strong.

One message for a future mum who had been trying to conceive for many years revealed that they were not 'coming in on a healing contract'. This beautiful woman had experienced a devastating loss at a very young age and, totally unbeknownst to her, part of the energy surrounding her desperation for a baby was an attempt to fill the hole within her that this loss had created. Her future baby wanted her mum to recognise this loss, understand it, and through healing the trauma of it, fill up this hole with love herself.

## What's love got to do with it?

Love is, of course, a very common theme for spirit babies, and the babies wishing for their mums to see themselves as they see them – as pure love. For their mums to love themselves.

Why is this? Because apart from the fact that we're all here to find our way back to love and loving ourselves, all of who we are, how can we teach our children that they are worthy of love, that they are love? That they are powerful and have every right to speak their truth without fear, to be themselves and not spend their lives trying to conform and fit into somebody else's rules and opinions, if we are not doing that ourselves? There is no pressure or blame here; we are all doing the best with can with what we know at the time. We can offer our babies a different experience if we are no longer carrying old patterns and traumas from the mother wound down the line.

We may say the words because we want our children to feel they are loved and powerful, but children, especially these high-vibration children, will see through this immediately. Knowingly or unknowingly, they will be questioning their own self-worth and trusting their own knowing that they are love.

Our children mirror us. Up until the age of seven or so, we are in a hypnotic state, a theta brainwave literally downloading everything around us, not just words but actions, what is going on in our environment and importantly, the energy we are putting out.

Women often carry beliefs such as we are not 'allowed' to love ourselves, that this is embarrassing, shameful, showing off, and we should be meek and humble. These stem from the mother wound and beliefs passed down from generation to generation. Also, this skewed idea of power – that power is often interpreted as having power 'over', and therefore we don't want to be powerful. True power, I believe, is gentle, peaceful, a power that comes from having self-belief, nothing to prove, nothing to fear. Power to express yourself, use your voice, know you are worthy.

And, beautiful ladies, it stops here. These beliefs stop with you. If you read on through the chapters around the bigger, bigger picture and the collective, you will gain an insight into just how key your own healing is.

Your babies are offering you a gift. I know this may be truly difficult to get your head around, especially when you have been waiting for so long, and doing everything you could possibly think of to get it right, or struggling with loss. But in the waiting is a gift, in the loss is a gift, the gift of self-discovery. Find yourself, find us is a consistent message from these incredible spirit babies.

## What gifts is your baby offering you? A note on the gift from Rosa

The gift upon gifts that your babies are offering you. For we know that they do not feel like gifts. These gifts of loss, of abandonment, these gifts of loneliness and grief and unworthiness.

Yet we see it differently. We see it as a gift of self-awareness, a gift of healing. As each woman rises through the pain of loss to see to the other side of it, they will see their very own baby spirits staring right back at them.

They will see their very own baby spirits being exactly what they have and always will be – their love, their gift – no matter whether that be here in person or in spirit. For there are very many gifts on this journey to motherhood.

The bitterness and the bile that can arise from a lost loved one or one who has been waiting for many years for their baby to arrive. And their baby may well be saying: "not yet, for I am not ready. I also can see that you are not ready. The bitterness and anger that my journey with you has brought up has not come from this journey with me but from a journey perhaps earlier in this lifetime or even another. It is this gift we offer you, that we are offering you as you grieve for us and wait for us. The gift of seeing all of this that lies within you that you truly no longer need to be holding as you lift yourselves ever more higher and higher towards the light."

For this is what your Soul wishes to do: lift higher and higher out of the energies of the mud, the doom and gloom, the guilt, heartache, anger and blame; the loss and the resentment, the hard done by and the victim.

For you are none of these things.

You are women of light. You have chosen and been chosen to be women of light. And so you must be true to yourselves as holders and carriers of the light to first clear the way through all of these lower resentments and energies in order for you to not only see yourselves as light and carriers of light – but be the carrier of light that we agreed upon with you oh so many moons ago.

We wish you well our beautiful, courageous women of light, for we know this is far from an easy journey. We too had to experience the loss of the light in our lifetimes in order for us to realise that we are indeed the light. And we wish you well on your journeys to see your light, feel it and embrace it, and to welcome the gifts of your babies here in spirit, whether they are to return or not.

They are always with you and always by your side on your journey ever more out of the darkness and into the true light of yourselves. It is to them that they will come, in droves and masses that you have never seen the like of before.

So please accept our love and please accept our gifts for we have nothing but love for you and this is all we wish you to see.

So just as you can imagine yourselves waking us up gently from our slumbers when we finally reach your world, so too this is what we are asking of you; that you too are awakening from your own slumbers and your own pain in order to see the light that is you and the light that is in front of you, for always.

If anyone had said to me 'what a gift', after I'd experienced any of my miscarriages, I'd have either crumpled in a heap or punched them in the face! Now I can see the gifts, I'm so grateful for the gifts that my journey to motherhood and as a mother bring me. However, we each get to that place in our own time of healing. Being so kind to yourself, allowing yourself to receive support if you can, finding someone who can help you understand at whatever level you're ready to, feel better and find peace with your experience is paramount. At some point in time, when you're ready, you'll begin to feel the gift. Until that time, please know you're held in love, your babies are with you and the gifts are waiting for whenever you're ready to receive them.

Reading this book so far, I hope you're beginning to know and feel that you are not on this journey alone, that your baby, too, is making their own choices about the who, the when, and the how. Add in a bit of divine timing and it really is a miracle that any babies are born at all! But each and every woman and each and every baby have their own unique path in this – together. Birth is a miracle, babies are miracles, a little piece of heaven coming into earth, and you, you are the miracle too. You too had to go through the process your spirit babies are now going through. You were the miracle baby, and you still are the miracle, the miracle woman, the miracle mother and miracle creator.

The souls coming in, and waiting to come in, want to hit the ground running. Therefore they need parents to be awake and aware. Parents who understand that their babies are souls in their own right with their own plans and life purpose, and that they need to be given the freedom to explore and express who they are. Parents who will support and guide them on their paths from this place of understanding, from this place of love. And for that, we need to first love and understand ourselves.

Your babies in spirit are showing tremendous courage and bravery in coming into the world at this time in order to heal it, just as you did. They are of a very high loving vibration and light and need their parents to feel the same way.

And this is the same for children already here. It is never too late to begin your inner journey to transform not only your life but that of your children.

**Rosa's message with a request from the future babies:**

> Do not fear, my little ones, for your little ones are with me and they are well. There are many, many baby spirits here with me. I wish to let you know that all is well. That your loss

is part of a grand plan that is yet to be revealed to you. Do not fear, because it will be when the time is right.

There are many, many babies here waiting for you to bring them into form, waiting to be welcomed, waiting to be loved, waiting for you to show yourselves as the true parents you are, parents who will love, honour, and respect them for the spirits that they are.

My message is, do not fear, for if you feel them in your space, or you feel you are a mum already, then this is indeed the case for they are with you and letting you know that.

Trust that, believe that, no matter what is going on for you, for they are here, of that I assure you. They are playing and they are gathering and they are waiting. So decide now whether it is them that you truly want, or whether there is something stopping you from welcoming them in.

They are asking that you are a pure soul who needs only to give and receive love from them and who will allow them to succeed in their own tasks and perhaps not the ones that you wish them to succeed in.

Maybe some will be doctors and lawyers, but there may also be some who simply wish to live their lives with a more quiet introspection that will change the way the world is done.

It is important not to hold any expectations of the when or the how or the who. It is only important to feel their love and allow them to do the rest. For they know what they want and they know what they are here to do.

What we must do is allow them that freedom and that choice in order that their wishes may be fulfilled. I cannot say this enough or more clearly: they have their own paths that you must agree to in order for them to agree and feel comfortable coming to you.

It is unconditional love that is needed here and for that to take place you must first look to the love that you feel for yourself. For without this love of yourself, how will you be able to show them the way – the way that is right and honourable for them?

For all they know now will be locked inside. Your role is to help them find the key to unveil and unravel to them their very essence and their very heart and the very truth of themselves in order that they may shine and reveal to themselves what they are here for.

And this message is to all parents, whether they are with child, have child, or wish to be with child. See your essence and you will help them to see theirs. And so it is with my blessings and the blessings and wishes of your babies here in spirit.


Ask yourself on a scale of zero to ten – ten being completely true – how much do I love myself? Do this without judgement, it's just a number where you're at. It's from here, all things can change.

# Chapter 9
## Learning to Love Ourselves
### Why are we so hard on ourselves and how to transform negative thoughts

Why is it so hard to love ourselves, or even, sometimes, to be kind to ourselves?

Life has a way of throwing all sorts of things at us that can seemingly knock us off course and stop us from seeing ourselves as love. Sometimes culturally, particularly for women, loving yourself, admiring yourself, knowing yourself to be a powerful, beautiful woman inside and out, standing up and out as your self, is not deemed acceptable, normal or appropriate. Apart from in this lifetime, the suppression and control of women has gone on for eons. We will be looking at this more closely in the second part of this book.

In this lifetime, many experiences can make us feel disempowered and hold us back from loving ourselves or feeling worthy of love. There are the bigger moments such as birth trauma (your own or your child's), childhood trauma, sexual assault and abuse, loss and bullying, as well as the less intense but no less impactful traumas that leave a sense of helplessness. They all add to feelings of not being safe, not being worthy, not being able to love or be loved.

Our families, teachers, leaders, and the media can all play a part – knowingly or unknowingly – telling us what we 'should' be and how we 'should' be, what is right and what is wrong, to the point where we no longer know who we are or what we believe about ourselves or the world. The messages from Rosa and other spirit beings tell us that it is time to clear space in our hearts and minds, to become really clear on who we are, what is our truth, and what we are holding onto that is not ours. What beliefs and opinions have we taken on board that don't belong to us and which ones are potentially holding us back from becoming a mum?

One of the key points in Rosa's messages is that we need to love and believe in ourselves – full stop.

These babies coming in are of such a high vibration they need to know and be reassured that they have your full support and guidance as their parents in order to help them remember they are love and deserving of love. If you do not love yourself, how will they know how to love themselves? If you are hoping a baby will fill you with the love that you're looking for, what lesson are you teaching them here about their own power and love? Quite apart from the pressure a baby, and indeed anyone you are in relationship with, may feel to provide you with this.

This is the same for each and every person, and in this context especially so for parents and those who have chosen the role of grandmother, aunty, sister, or best friend of these mums, as well as guides for these children of light in the form of nannies, teachers, and counsellors.

The spirit babies need to know they have your support, your understanding, your blessing. They need to feel safe enough, special enough, to show up in the world as themselves and not feel like they have to fit into society to people-please or because they're scared, but instead create the society in which they wish to live.

So the question is: why is it so hard to believe in yourself; to believe you'll be a mum? I invite you to step outside of the pain for a moment and ask yourself what is it that your journey so far is showing you? What is it offering you?

It is clear there is a real need for us all to know ourselves, who we are, and to clear away all the mind chatter and terrible stories we tell ourselves about ourselves. All those negative thoughts and beliefs and the energy they bring with them. It's a time for clarity, a deeper understanding, and trust.

Spirit, and your babies in spirit, is asking you to know yourself and ultimately know yourself as love so you can hold the light that they are bringing and trust that you will guide them in their mission.

When it comes to talking to doctors about miscarriage and infertility, the terms used are unexplained miscarriage or unexplained infertility. I believe there is always an explanation, however. Much of this lies within ourselves. There is the physical and health aspect of course, which isn't covered in this book, but our mindset and emotional aspect are also key.

The stress of living in a modern world and the effects of stress on our body and the balance of hormones is a key area to explore first. There are the well-known and accepted ways of reducing stress by taking physical action such as creating a better work/life balance, diet, meditation, mindfulness, yoga and other exercise.

Another way to reduce stress is to go a bit deeper into our minds and emotional states. Our mind, body, and soul hold onto our life traumas – our own experiences and the beliefs, largely unconscious ones, that we made about ourselves and the world because of them. These can span back to our own time in the womb and our own births – and, of course, from lives before.

By becoming aware of how these traumas and beliefs affect our bodies and our opportunity to become pregnant, we have the potential to transform them. We can change the way we think and feel about ourselves through energy healing practices.

## Changing negative beliefs

Let's move out of the higher realms for a moment and into the physical realm to look briefly at what is going on here in this world, in this time and space, that may be preventing you from meeting with your baby. What is causing your stress, your anxiety? What is causing you to feel low and to speak to yourself, and treat yourself, unkindly?

Essentially, what is stopping you from seeing yourself as love?

It is so important to realise it is not the external situation that's causing your suffering. It's your thoughts about the situation that are causing your suffering. Does that make any sense right now? It's tough, as then it's almost impossible to apportion blame for your ills.

Blaming our pain on the past, someone else or something else, is a way of distancing ourselves from having to take responsibility in the here and now to heal ourselves.

A harsh but brave and necessary lesson at going within.

On our journeys to motherhood, there are very many uncomfortable buttons within us that are pushed. There can be a great sense of failure, of guilt, grief and shame, a why-me, victim-type energy that can show itself. Anger, bitterness and resentment can be constant companions no matter how much we try to stifle them and think them away.

Have you ever wondered why? Have these feelings suddenly appeared because of what you're going through now or was there another time, another situation, where they came up?

Here is a quick exercise to highlight the mind/body connection. Close your eyes and imagine there is a tray of juicy lemons in front of you. You choose one and cut it in half. You're now going to imagine smelling that lemon. Now you're going to imagine eating that lemon – rind and all. You can feel the lemon juice saturate your tongue and trickle down your throat. Is your mouth watering? Is your face screwing up? In most cases, when people imagine eating the lemon, they experience an increased production of saliva.

This happens because we have a memory of what a lemon tastes like, and our physiology responds to that memory. This is a simple connection to make – your mind remembers the lemon and your body responds, even when the lemon isn't real.

Most often our subconscious reactions to a situation or a word is not such a straightforward connection and almost impossible to logically think through. As an example, from the moment I had Max, I used to become really stressed every time he needed to sleep. I thought this was normal. I was desperate for him to sleep, needed him to sleep, so I could rest. But this feeling went on and on right through to when my second son Samuel was four years old. Ten years of bedtime stress.

Max being Max, a gentle, self-contained little soul, meant it barely had an effect. Samuel, on the other hand, is a different matter. He seriously was pushing my buttons at bedtime to the point where I finally knew I had to address it. And so I set about using the healing technique known as EFT tapping. EFT stands for Emotional Freedom Technique.

The tapping brought the most incredible rage and anger to the surface to the point of being quite frightening. I wondered where it was taking me.

It took me to a memory of my four-year-old self about to be 'put to sleep' for a heart operation. I was terrified. I thought I was being attacked, killed, and I had no power whatsoever to do anything about it. It may sound utterly bonkers but putting my own children 'to sleep' was firing up my subconscious mind to that memory and sending me right back into all of the stress, fear and emotions of my four-year-old self.

I drew on all my energy healing tools, including Theta, colour healing, angel healing, Matrix Reimprinting, and the techniques of EFT, founded by Karl Dawson, to change it. I helped and healed my little self, empowered her to change how she felt about what was going on. In so doing, we changed the energy around that situation which eradicated the emotional charge

And bedtime changed.

Samuel had been reacting to my own energy of stress – a clear example of how our children, and in fact, anyone around us, is affected by what is going on with ourselves. It also demonstrates what powerful teachers our little ones are as they push those buttons that need pushing so we bring attention to what's going on inside ourselves that needs healing. Another reason why you can't separate your journey to motherhood from your soul journey – because it continues when your children are here in the world.

# Why do we feel and respond the way we do?

I believe in the statement that our children are our greatest teachers. This is the same in my eyes whether you are physically with your child, they chose not to stay, or are yet to be born. There is no real linear explanation as to why we feel what we feel, or think what we think. But we are energy, and if we follow the energy, starting with the most pressing issue, most often with the support of a trained practitioner, and delving into our subconscious mind, we can find the answers and transform the limiting beliefs and feelings.

If we take responsibility for our own healing, we are not only helping ourselves, but all of those around us. Subconscious reactions can also be triggered by particular words, because words carry a meaning and the body responds to that meaning. For me, these words were putting to sleep.

One little girl, whose mum had recently had a miscarriage, suddenly became terrified of going to school and being away from her mum. It transpired that this little girl had heard her mum talking about 'losing' the baby. This little girl was terrified her mum might lose her too.

As adults, we understand the context and have a lot more life experience to make sense of things. However, as children, our minds work very differently. Thankfully, this little girl's fear was addressed immediately, and hopefully, that fear of being lost won't follow her into adulthood. However, many of us are still carrying childhood traumas that can affect how our lives are running now.

What is going on in our minds, totally without us knowing, can create stress and a physiological reaction that can inhibit the release of the hormones we need to become pregnant.

The amygdala – that little almond-shaped group of cells or nuclei in your brain – is the first part to form and is part of the limbic system. It is often called our reptilian brain as it deals with our most basic needs for survival.

The amygdala controls the flight, fight, or freeze response. If you have a fear of heights, for example, whether you are physically up high, seeing a picture, or even just imagining being up high, the effect is the same. Your limbic system will kick in, blood will rush from your thinking brain, your digestive system, and your reproductive system – you don't need to think or eat or reproduce when you are faced with danger – and flood your respiratory system as your muscles prepare you to run or fight.

We need this response to keep us safe from danger and to react quickly to a potential accident. Even when it comes to an event that should actually be quite pleasant – a party, a holiday, a telephone call, making love – our minds will flick through the files, picking out the last time a similar event happened, and if it didn't go too well for some reason, your mind will try and protect you by going into a stress response of flight, fight, or freeze.

Any decisions made in that moment of 'trauma' are subject to your mind starting to look for evidence of the belief that it's not safe. Seek and you shall find! So we need to keep all the innate responses, such as knowing not to jump off a cliff, jumping out of the way of a car, and reacting to danger, but turn off all the false, programmed reactions.

Our minds are incredible and most of our stress triggers are buried deep, deep down in a place we're not even aware of.

And this is why. The conscious mind – the thinking part that works out a new route to somewhere, figures out the new computer programme, learns how to wire a plug – the part that deals with logic, is responsible for about 5 to 15 percent of our brain, depending on the studies you look at.

The subconscious runs the remaining 85 to 95 percent. This is the part that allows you to never forget how to ride a bike or drive your car – or even drive your car home without you actually remembering how you got to your regular destination because it has been hard-wired as a deeply ingrained 'habit'.

When you make a decision to go on a diet, or go running every day, or become pregnant, whatever it may be – the decisions you make such as: I will be a mum, I will not eat that cake, I will go to the gym, I will be nice to my boss, I won't be angry about this or resentful about that, I will go through that IVF cycle without worry – using your conscious mind, your willpower, to achieve your goal is just about the hardest uphill struggle. It's your old Nokia going up against NASA's supercomputer.

The supercomputer is your subconscious mind – your hard drive – the back end of your computer kicking in. All those things you've learnt in life from conception – and before.

## What effect does this have on conception?

In terms of your journey to motherhood, your conscious mind and every bit of you is screaming yes, yes, yes, of course I want to be a mum, but running on the bigger computer may be programmes such as: I'm not good enough. It's dangerous. Will I be a good mum? What if I'm like my mum? What if my partner leaves me?

We tell ourselves: I'm too old to get pregnant; I partied too hard; being a mum is hard; I'll be a rubbish mum; I don't deserve it; I did something bad and I deserve to be punished; I have this diagnosis so it's unlikely I can get pregnant; I won't be able to cope; it will be too much; I'm scared of giving birth.

We are mostly totally unaware of those beliefs running in the background, that we're running a programme that says: life is a struggle, I have to fight for what I want; the world is dangerous (and therefore too dangerous for my baby).

Or there are fears and decisions you made based on your own past traumas. There may have been miscarriage loss; there may have been a termination or abuse and you don't feel safe. If you don't feel safe, do you feel you are a 'safe' home for your baby to come into?

We are conscious beings in the womb and if your mum was in any way stressed, or experienced grief or a shock, for example, whilst she was pregnant with you, this may have been seen as a threat to your own survival and a decision made buried deep in your foetal subconscious that is affecting you now.

I only very recently found out that I was a womb twin. Doing what I do, I've picked this up quite a number of times for my clients and it's more common than I realised, certainly for those who find me to work with. Some are aware they were a twin, but like me, it came as a bit of a shock and a revelation to understand why they were feeling certain emotions, feeling loss, abandonment, or that a part of them was missing.

But despite all the work around my own birth, this particular aspect had never come up. It did when I was exploring the feeling I had of always having something missing, a hole to fill, as well as bigger feelings of loss and also betrayal. With my own spiritual mentor, I was taken back into the womb and unexpectedly met my womb twin, a little boy who had chosen not to stay. I discovered he came in with me to 'hold my hand' during the enormity of coming into earth but was never meant to stay. He is now one of my guides and works in the Christ light energy of unconditional love – New Earth energy.

This is why going back to our own birth stories, for everyone but certainly as mums-in-waiting, I believe, is key. You need to identify any experiences you had as a baby in the womb that may be running some sort of programme telling you that it's not safe out there. Clearing any trauma from your own birth also helps to ensure history doesn't repeat itself when you give birth to your own child. It shouldn't, but it still amazes me when women who come to me suffering with birth trauma reveal they had a similar birth experience to their child's. This is the power of our subconscious mind, constantly reminding us through our experiences of what is laying there calling to be healed.

We often have more of an incentive for our own health when trying to become pregnant, but if you're running programmes of comforting yourself with food, for example, this is going to put extra pressure on you – you'll be in conflict with yourself and therefore in stress.

All of these beliefs can throw you into that stress response. My saying that has likely triggered you, so put your hand on your heart and breathe gently in for six and out for six.

Energy-healing tools allow you to release those fears that either come from the past or from projecting yourself into the future. They all feel very real but I can assure you that they are not. This is stuck energy, which can be moved and shifted.

Add in the spiritual element (everything being spiritual simply because we are), and I've found that the mums and mums-in-waiting now also have the bigger task of healing ancestral patterns for their female line going back in time and into the future. This is not limited to us women, men also have agreed on soul level to address ancestral trauma, much as my own did. So you are not only healing yourself with this work, you are healing far more than you can imagine.

We have all taken on the beliefs and realities of others. As the film, Good Will Hunting with Robin Williams and Matt Damon says, 'It's not your fault'. There was little you could do as a child, but there is plenty you can do now.

We are all individually responsible for ourselves. However, at some soul level, you chose to take on those beliefs, which brings us to the bigger picture – there's always a bigger picture! On a more philosophical level, this is life, and our challenges and our beliefs are the very things we are here to overcome in order to grow as people.

Let's look at an anecdote of three brothers. Their father wasn't a very nice person. He told them all they would amount to nothing. The first boy did just that and struggled with life. The second boy took on this belief but had an inspiring teacher who encouraged him and told him how good he was and about the potential he had. This brother went through life with an inner battle between these two beliefs – I'm no good; I am good – and each time he succeeded, he often sabotaged his own success. The third brother succeeded in everything he did. He chose not to take on his father's words and chose not to absorb them.

So you see: we all choose our individual paths. And these later become our opportunities. Your journey to motherhood is one of those opportunities, a gift from your babies, to help you, and often jolt you in what doesn't seem the best of ways. Our job is to start looking within; to start discovering who we truly are, by peeling back the layers and programmes built up in life.

We are bombarded with life, ours and everyone else's we come into contact with, from the moment of conception, as well as from what we bring in with us. This could be a trauma carried over from a past life that you've brought back in order to heal. A lot of my clients end up somewhere other than in this lifetime and it's always illuminating and extremely powerful healing.

The power of our thoughts cannot be underestimated. What we put out there – knowingly or unknowingly – the universe gives us back.

If you are desperately 'wanting' a baby, you remain in that energy of wanting. My wish for you is that if your wish is to become a mum, this book might move you from the waiting room and into the happening room. Because the moment you begin to look within and take action to change the energy you are putting out into the world, is the moment the universe responds.

It may be worth jotting down a few of your most common thoughts about yourself. In one column write the thought, look at it, say it out loud over and over and ask yourself: is that true? In the next column, write down a more positive thought. This exercise is a great way of looking at your thoughts and fears and flipping your mindset. You can also bring the candle flame exercise in from earlier too to help dissolve them. Or it may be time to find a qualified energy healer you're drawn to, to support you in making sense of your thoughts and beliefs and any underlying trauma that created them.

## What has age got to do with it?

A common belief for many of my clients, who are in their late thirties and forties or have reached their 50 milestone, is 'I'm too old'. I remember, at 37, being pregnant with Max and described in medical terms as a geriatric mother – what! What kind of language is that? How would that make any new mum feel? It is, in my opinion, disgusting and another example of the age-old patriarchy controlling a women's body. Along with failed cycle and labour, the terms alone makes you feel like you're going into battle and exhausted before you begin. Similarly, moments in labour when they use terms such as failure to progress, or incompetent cervix. The blame and responsibility of 'failure' are always put on the woman. What effect is this language going to have on a woman who is at both her most powerful and vulnerable? Seriously, no more! How about we start with a change of language that is more empowering to women?

Luckily, I didn't have that programme running of I'm too old and could laugh at it. And, of course, I had Samuel when I was 42. I know so many, many women who are mums in their late forties and aged 50.

One of the bravest, most beautiful and gifted women I've been honoured to meet is Karen, a natural and intuitive healer. From a young age, Karen knew she wanted to be a mum. She felt her babies around her from her twenties. However, with the way life works, and the curveballs it can throw at you, Karen married a man who was already a dad and didn't want any more children.

Throughout some difficult marital times, Karen felt and saw her babies, which led to confusion. If what she felt and saw was real, how was it to happen? It took some time for Karen to find her voice and her power within this relationship and the strength to say 'yes' to her dreams. She walked away. Her journey to motherhood then took a very different turn as potentially a single mum. Karen did not lose hope in her dream. She felt her babies around her and knew that this is what she was meant to do.

Her healing journey towards motherhood was a very long and difficult fifteen years of health problems, IVF cycles, egg donation, and miscarriage. She had begun to lose trust in her own intuition about 'seeing' her babies, when she re-connected with one of her former Reiki pupils, now a channel, spiritual teacher and healer,

Olwen Jennings. Karen was able to talk directly to Olwen's guides about why she hadn't yet had a successful pregnancy and whether she should keep trying. It was very clear from the very first session with Olwen that she should keep trying as there was a very special soul waiting to be birthed. In fact, the soul of this baby came through with Olwen's guides and Olwen was able to pass on messages from him.

This soul is highly evolved with a very high vibration. A soul who needed to come to earth to shine his light and help with Ascension. Ascension, as I see it, is clearing enough space in our energy by releasing the lower vibration energies such as resentment, guilt, grief, and jealousy so more of your soul light can come in. Ascension is actually a descending of your higher energies into the physical – bringing heaven down to earth.

This high soul had chosen Karen and needed her to do certain things, such as clearing energy blocks, stepping into her truth and her power, and to really prepare herself to carry him as he was so full of light. He chose Karen as she, too, is full of light and can give to him what he needs.

It was Olwen's guides who directed Karen to me for more specialist help. They were such beautiful, powerful sessions with the energy of Mother Mary very present. It wasn't long before insight came from Karen's own meditations, a channelled message from Rosa, and Olwen's guides, all confirming it was time for her to begin the process of her egg transfer, from sperm and egg donation. I'm still to this day and every day, in awe of Karen's resilience and trust in her intuition, her babies and the messages and signs from spirit to follow the guidance. Karen became pregnant. It was a pregnancy where she really needed to listen to her body and rest as much as possible and her son came earlier than expected – in time for the new moon and solar eclipse, of course!

On 30 June 2019, her son Oliver was born. Karen had just turned 51. I have met and cuddled with this very special little boy whom I'd met in his spirit form and, of course, shed a few tears of joy. Precious times, and I know that Karen, Oliver, and I will continue this beautiful friendship as he grows up and gives his mum the runaround!

That's the energy of miracles.

## Karen tells her story

I'm trying to work out how long this journey has been. The problems started in 2004. I wasn't in a good place with my marriage, but I had such powerful visions and connections to my spirit babies I kept going with it, hoping he would change his mind about children. We had a small spare room, which the previous owners had for their granddaughter. It had the same curtains as one of my nieces and it would have made a perfect nursery.

I had to take the curtains down and had some others made. I set it up to be a therapy room. I had hoped to start seeing Reiki clients again, but every time I went in that room, I'd feel upset and I then decided that if I couldn't help myself, how could I help others? I stopped my Reiki business. I would still send Reiki remotely and would often give courses at my parent's house, but depression set in. I kept asking the angels and Mother Mary and everyone else for help. There was a final straw that came when I finally left my husband. All through these difficult times my little angel would appear before me, so I hung on, but although I couldn't see how I could be a mum to them physically, I just knew I would be.

At first, I had a vision of a boy and a girl. Then the soul would come to me as a female, called Trinity. She occasionally appeared with her twin soul, Luna. Trinity appeared with dark hair and Luna with blonde. On the whole, it was mainly the one soul. I then started seeing a massive blue light and knew it was my child. There was a distinct male energy to the blue orb and I would sadly go along to Mothercare and buy something for the future and thought how mad that was. A psychic friend would always say I'd have a boy, but I gave up listening and thought she'd got it wrong. How wrong was I!

The stories of the soul and that part of the journey are so long I could write a book about it myself. I've rarely spoken about Trinity and someone once suggested that Trinity might have to be born in male form to complete the mission they would be born to do. I kept thinking I was going mad, but the soul I now know as Oliver kept making his presence known with this blue light and a strong energy.

I always knew, even years before, that I had to keep going so that I could bring my little one into this world. I came across the book by Walter Makichen (Spirit Babies: How to Communicate with the Child You're Meant to Have) and everything changed. It made me see that I wasn't mad and that babies chose their parents and how they arrived, whether naturally or through medical intervention. I had to keep going despite everything; something, this little soul, was urging me forward. I gave up so many times but never really gave up as each time I was given another nudge and another sign they were coming.

I first saw an advert on the tube for a fertility clinic and went along for a talk in December 2013, a couple of months after separating from my husband. I booked an appointment that day for January and that was the start of it all: 2014 until now. I naively thought it would just be an insemination, but Oliver had other plans. At the time all was well with me physically in terms of eggs but then through life stress, it became clear I would need to be going down both the egg and sperm donation route.

I had already chosen the male donor for an IUI in 2014 that hadn't been successful, but I had now gone past the date of using them again so I had to choose all over again. This didn't feel too difficult at the time; it was the whole egg donor issue that upset me the most, and it took me more or less a year to get my head around that. Having now read about spirit babies, however, it made it easier to deal with the egg donor situation, as I was seeing it through the eyes of my future child. Their soul had chosen to come this way, a bit of one person, a bit of another, but had chosen me to be his or her mummy. I could get upset that I was going it alone, or that the baby wouldn't be genetically mine, but knowing that this is what the soul had chosen, and that this was the only way, helped me get through it and move forwards. In December 2015 I decided to go ahead and start IVF with the egg and sperm donors.

The whole of 2016 was taken up with IVF, pushing my body through three embryo transfers. I had started treatment in the December of 2015 and went right through to December 2016 with four IVF treatments. I went abroad to my parents and I was in a total mess. I had started to have a reaction to the steroids and I was all puffed up. My hair started falling out too and I was physically and emotionally drained.

I changed clinics in 2017 and had to sign up with the egg donor agency pretty quickly due to their age cut-off point. My forty-ninth birthday was in three weeks, and I would have been too old to sign up with them as they had changed the cut-off age by about three years. It took them most of the year to find the donor I ended up with. I had one failed IVF cycle and then a mock cycle to check the timing of the transfers and that involved a biopsy of my uterus.

I then decided to give myself a break and take a rest from it all. I was at my limit, but still, I couldn't give up. I changed my diet and reconnected with one of my Reiki students, Olwen, who was now channelling her guides. It was Olwen's guides who suggested I begin working with Debra. Between us all, the healing, the guidance and the messages, it became clear that November 2018 was the time. I finally had the last transfer on 6 November 2018. I felt Rosa's energy with me.

And here we are. I'm a mum, a tired mum right now, sometimes a little stressed mum, but a mum to this beautiful soul whom I never gave up on and who never gave up on me. My darling Oliver was meant to be and meant to arrive just the way he is.

Please hold the light of your miracle. Sending love to you all.

Karen's story, her faith and belief that part of her purpose was to receive and hold the light of the fabulous Oliver as we now know him, inspires me every day. So sure of their love and connection, Karen kept going despite some truly horrible, heartbreaking and stressful times. Karen felt comforted by the spiritual perspective that our babies have a choice in who and how they wish to arrive and you may wish to go back to this earlier chapter on why IVF or egg donation is a choice.

Fellow spirit baby medium, Kelly Meehan, who actually created the term, Spirit Baby Medium, and who also powerfully supports women and couples on their conception journey, kept relaying to Karen from her spirit baby we now know as Oliver that Karen had to go deeper, go deeper into herself.

I was honoured to play my part in the journey with Karen and Oliver that held them in the energies of the Divine Mother and guided Karen inwards to heal, clear out the lower energies of trauma, betrayal and disempowerment, and gain insight and self-belief. When you do this you make room for and allow space in your body and energy for more of the higher vibration energies of love and joy. This is ascension – more of your higher soul light, descending into your physical body here on earth. And, of course, Oliver embodies the energies of love and joy.

The second of Karen's spirit babies was such a powerful soul. When I asked why I could hear her but not feel her, her response was to laugh with glee and say she'd blow my socks off if she allowed me to feel her – such is her high vibration. And we wait to see where her story unfolds now in either this earth or another realm, as one of Karen's and Oliver's guides perhaps.

After reading Karen's magical story, it seems a little vacuous to come down and talk about age. Karen felt judged for trying to become a mum at 50. Luckily, her fertility clinic didn't buy into that and was very supportive. Karen was strong enough and had enough belief in herself and her babies to rise above this conditioning and fear of judgement to do what was right for her – an incredible gift in healing the mother wound. Since Karen, two more women in their fifties, whom I have been honoured to serve, are now mums to three babies in total, and I'm sure another on the way.

Like most things, it is what you believe that matters. Below is a very interesting, mind-blowing message from Melchizedek on ageing. Keep an open mind on this one. It certainly got me thinking about how conditioning plays a role in what we think life should be and about what's possible!

Mostly, holding onto the thought I'm too old is a belief. If you are running it, because that is our culture right now, it can be released – it is not the truth of who you are.

Melchizedek is a high priest who is mentioned in the Bible's book of Genesis. His role is to help us all with raising our vibration – lifting us back to a state of love and oneness and assisting the earth through the ascension process, whereby low-vibration energies are cleared away to allow the light of the soul to come in.

## Message from Melchizedek on age

We can also offer you and all of your many readers some of the realities of the body. For just as you are all a part of the all and everything, so too are your cells and molecules and atoms, and so too must they be loved as the universe loves them and loved by you for all they do and all they share out into the world. For do you see that just as the energy of the universe never ceases, neither does the energy of your cells? The energy of your cells must be fuelled equally as the universe is fuelled, for they are one and the same thing.

And can you imagine the universe ever dying through lack of energy? So why then can you envisage the cells in your body dying? Is it because at heart you all wish to give up this life on earth and actually come home to us here in the ethers?

For surely if you wished to stay and remain then you would be believing that you, as a part of a never-ending, never-dying universe, don't have to die either – ever. So we are asking you to see your cells and treat your cells as you treat the universe, for that is indeed what they are.

To see these cells of yours as never-ending or never-dying and yet instead as ever-expanding and ever-living. Ever-changing indeed and yet never ceasing to be. So can you see how this change in perception may bring about a longer life? And can you see how this change in perception can bring about a more full life and one that you know you are in control of and indeed not at the mercy of what you call the ageing process?

For indeed the universe is ageing and changing, but at the same time it is not, it simply is. This is the same for you. Do not succumb to the notion that you must die in order to live. Or die in order to return to us here in the higher heavens, for the point is, my dear, you are already in and already are that higher heaven.

## Afraid of dying or afraid of living?

There is no reason to die and there is no reason to age except for the belief that this is so. So, my dear, you can tell these women, and indeed tell these men, that there is no such thing as the ageing process and there is only the thing of wishing to die, and therefore altering the cells to no longer function as optimally as they can, in order for this to happen.

And this would be a shame for the many who would like to live and a shame for the many who have long waited to see this statement of bringing heaven to earth, because do you see, my dear, it is in fact one and the same thing?

So do not choose to die. Do not choose for your cells to die for this is only an example of you missing 'home' and missing 'us' when in fact we are already here and you are already home. This may well be a big concept for you to understand and certainly, there will be many who simply choose not to believe, and the only reason for this is that they are choosing not to stay. Choosing not to stay in this body or in this lifetime for they feel so far away from home that they cannot bear to be apart from it for so long. And yet you, my dear, now know differently and so you too can choose right here and right now to live or to die and to start all over again.

You can surely come back here at any time, whether it is you who chooses to come back here through a passing of time on earth, or whether you come back through the imaginations of your mind, for truly this is all just one and the same thing.

Your body my dear, does not need to age, as the cells are the cells of the universe, ever-changing and ever-expanding, and ever experiencing different stages, and yet never going anywhere completely out into the nothingness. For the nothingness is already here within you too.

Set your sights on living, my dear, and set your sights on loving your cells and being with your cells just as you are setting your sights on loving the universe and being with the universe for it truly is one and the same thing and once you know this, then it is surely time for others to know this.

Look after your bodies and your bodies will look after you, this is the exact same meaning as look after your earth and your earth will look after you. And look after your love and your love will look after you, the love of this being, of course, the love of the universe.

So when your women of light come to you to question just how it is they can become pregnant when they have reached a certain age in your human years, you can tell them that this concept is of course of no consequence unless they believe it to be so.

## Trust

Another major factor in how we experience life and our journeys to motherhood is how much we trust ourselves. Trust has been a huge learning curve for me and my own spiritual challenge in terms of my soul plan. However, as I mentioned near the beginning of this book, because of all my baby losses, and despite having every rational reason not to trust that my pregnancy with Samuel would go smoothly, I did have trust in my body. I was amazed and had to keep checking that I really was in trust because trusting felt so alien to me. But trust I did.

You heard from Karen how her trust in the messages she was receiving from her babies and from spirit kept her going, even through times when she didn't trust her body or herself.

Through my own experience, and through those of clients, I've come to realise that when we don't trust – trust ourselves, the universe, others – it is because of trauma and pain that remains in the body, that causes a disconnection. It's important to delve into this energy of mistrust by asking where does it come from? Who or what brought you into this place of mistrust? By resolving the situation or situations that have created mistrust, you can more easily move back into trust when life kicks you out of it. It's easier to re-find your centre.

**This message from Rosa offers a spiritual perspective on trust after loss.**

> My darling scribe, what is there not to trust? Does the sun not rise each day? Does the wind not blow? Do the flowers not grow? Does the sun not shine and the moon look sublime each and every day of your lives?
>
> And so, why not the trust? For you do not even question the trust that the earth will continue to turn, for it is not of your consequence, and it is not of your power, and it is not of your lives, or so you wish to think.
>
> Yet when something happens to make you think it is of your consequence, think it is of your power, even think it is your fault – it is then that you begin to question the trust. The trust in yourself and, of course, your trust in others, in life and the universe.

But do you not see there is no difference in trusting the turning of the earth, and the lack of worry this gives you, than the turning of the universe – your universe – from one of calm and flow to perhaps one of chaos?

It is in this chaos that you must remain in trust – for there really is no other way. It is not lack of trust in the universe here that is the issue. It is a lack of trust in yourself, a lack of faith in how you have come to this place of mistrust.

It is not trust that you should be looking to, but to the suffering that this situation of mistrust has brought you, whether that is the suffering of your mind, body or soul – this is where your focus should be. Not the suffering of not trusting, for there is no more you can do to make the world turn than what you are already doing – and that is having faith in yourself. Do you see the world is still turning, even when you do not have faith in yourself?

Why do you think this is? It is because we have you, and we hold you, and we honour you in love at all times and in all ways. We do not for one moment question the faith or question the trust that we have in you. We are simply asking the same in return – for you to see that trust within yourself that you will keep the world turning, and when it is you feel you cannot, then to know that this is what we and others are doing for you until you can resume your state of faith.

You will never be out of trust for long, for something else will surely happen to signal to you that your loved ones are indeed still at one with you, albeit from a different place, but with you nonetheless.

There is no changing of, or manipulation of, the universal laws – for they are simply the laws. Not laws to restrict, but laws to allow the life and the plan and the love of the universe to flow in full concert of what is meant to be. So why not have trust?

Why not have trust in the process of creation and this trust in the laws and in yourself? As I have said, this is nothing to do with trust, for once you all did live in full trust, no matter what the outward circumstances.

However, this was not to say that there was no heartbreak. And this was not to say there were no tears, sadness, or grief – but what there was not, were questions about integrity or questions around trust, because there was simply a time when just as you do not understand or have a play in the turning of the earth now, neither did you have to question anything about the events of the past. You simply knew it was meant to be for some reason.

The reason you were able to do this was because you were all connected, fully connected to the universal flow of life in which souls are souls with no beginning and no end. Souls are souls who can come and go and be and do entirely as their souls choose to come and go and be and do and entirely of their own desires and wishes for what is best for them at that time and not at the wishes of anyone else.

For they are not beholden to anyone else and neither, my dears, are you. So do not question your trust in what has happened. Perhaps it is time to explore why this happened for you in your lifetime, in this lifetime of yours.

## Connection leads to trust

I trust you will allow me to get to my point: that it is not the lack of trust that is the problem but the lack of connection which you feel. Connection to yourself, connection to the universe, connection to the flow of life, and, yes, your connection to your baby souls.

But please remember they are not simply your 'baby souls', but beautiful and powerful souls in their own right with their own choices and their own life plans – plans that indeed are very much linked to yours, but very much theirs alone too.

Can you trust your baby souls have made their right choices? Choices that are right for them, even if they feel so far from right for you? And can you trust that your own soul's calling is to have been a part, a very loving part, of this baby soul's journey thus far?

For once you can accept that there are no outcomes, no expectations, no holding onto, and no need to question the very turning of the universe, then we can actually turn to the pain this loss has delivered. The pain of ownership, the pain of control, the pain of losing the thoughts and expectations which you had placed upon these souls who have choice but to take their leave. And for you to question why this is so. For surely the loss of a child is the most grievous burn on a human soul, and it is only the bravest and most courageous who have offered to experience the pain of this burn.

For within this burn is always a new flourishing, a new seed, a new life than the one you ever thought possible. We are not saying this is an easy adjustment to make, but we are saying to please hold onto the burn of pain, turning and transforming into the most beautiful forest of love once again. A forest that may be very different from the one you once saw, but a forest nonetheless.

We hold you in our light as you move through the fire of pain and into the heat of the love and the light that lies beyond it – a world that is indeed very different, but one no less sublime and beautiful, than the one first imagined.

My dears, it is not a question of blame, of blaming your body, of blaming your diet, your beliefs, or even your 'self' or the universe, to the extent that you do not know how you will ever trust again.

Trust is innate – it is always there – it has simply been forgotten under the piles of pain. Yet within these piles are the secrets to life itself, and when you hold the secrets to life, you know there is no need to ever feel this or buy into this sense of mistrust ever again.

We ask you to resume within these moments of pain your connection with yourself and that which in turn is a connection to the entire universe.

And so it is.

With our love and blessings for your understanding of the complications in the simplicity that is life on your earth.

Sometimes all we can do is keep breathing and trusting. I'm not saying trust is easy, but when we can find this place of acceptance and trust, your world of possibility opens up. Not trusting highlights where there is unresolved trauma around a situation. By healing or easing any sense of trauma, you begin to feel able to trust yourself and where you're at. We're always told to trust and we may say it but it can create such a pressure when the truth is we don't. Maybe try a little EFT tapping on the word trust – be honest with yourself about not trusting and tap on the pressure you feel around this and it will ease. Reconnecting with yourself, your baby and Source, helps bring a sense of peace and trust that all will be okay.

Use the exercise of measuring from zero to ten – how much do you trust your body? your baby? that you'll become pregnant? Again, no judgement, it's just a number and numbers change. And then begin writing or meditating on where you feel this mistrust in your body. Make it tangible, give it a colour and a form. Ask how long it's been there and what it needs. Whatever the emotion that comes to mind which would help ease this sense of mistrust, ask what colour that emotion would be. Then bring in this new colour to your area of mistrust to help ease the energy.

## Healing beliefs

Before we move back in time and into the bigger picture of this book, your journey and your role in this picture, see below for a number of positive affirmations to help anything that may be hindering your own journey to motherhood. There are also others that are for general women's empowerment.

I have commanded distance healing on the below and invite you to simply say 'yes' to receiving the energy of these beliefs and allow that energy to move through you. The more we clear these unhelpful beliefs we hold knowingly or unknowingly, and bring in the more empowering ones, the lighter and stronger we feel and the more self-belief we hold. And with self-belief, we can do anything.

- I know what it feels like to be allowed to have children

- It's safe for me to have children

- My body is strong and functions perfectlyThe eggs in my body are strong

- I am ready for the child that is to be mine

- I am fertile

- I trust my partner will be a good father/parent

- I have enough love for everyone in my life

- I can love my partner and my baby

- With each passing day my body prepares for my baby

- My body is a perfect place for my baby to grow

- My body accepts my mate

- I have the highest truth and understanding of who I am

- I have the highest truth and understanding of my life purpose

- I know what it means and what it feels like to own my power

- I know what it feels like to be loved

- I know what it feels like to be love

- I know what it feels like to heal

- I know it is possible to heal

- I allow myself to, I deserve to, I am safe doing so, I know how to and I do live my life with this grace and ease now.

# Chapter 10
## Experiences that can keep us from Becoming a Mum
### Childhood Trauma, birth trauma, loss and termination

As with everything in life, experiences that may be holding you back from becoming a mum will be unique to each of you. Your own birth experience is a perfect place to start exploring beliefs, fears, and patterns that may be sending out the message 'it's not safe' to become pregnant, or 'it's painful being born', or you 'failed' at the very outset. There are so many patterns and beliefs that come from the way we ourselves were born.

Perhaps you were induced and therefore find it hard to make decisions for yourself, or you feel rushed or pushed into things. Or a forceps birth with your first experience of life being pain, being pulled, attacked even. All these traumas are stored in our subconscious minds and tend to pop up when we ourselves wish to create and birth life.

If you are already a mum and your birth experience was a shock, not what you expected, or very traumatic, this too can unknowingly be protecting you by not allowing the conditions to be right to conceive again, causing secondary infertility.

There are also, of course, all the biggies that I've mentioned previously: emotional and physical abuse, neglect and childhood trauma. A trauma that didn't have to be a huge trauma and may not seem or feel traumatic to our adult minds, however, to a child there may have been an event that created a deep wound. Maybe you accidentally hurt your sibling and were told off and told not to go near the baby – an experience of one of my clients.

Another of my clients experienced a great loss at a young age and the hole it left was understandably huge. Our babies are not coming in to heal our wounds – they are holding back from arriving, so you can heal your own wounds first. This beautiful lady's spirit baby was adamant they were not coming to heal her – that she needed to fill the absence with love for herself. And guess what? After a long and heartbreaking journey, she is now a mum to a very precious little boy.

One of the aspects I want to explore here in more depth is that of termination – or releasing your baby as I choose to refer to this deeply traumatic experience – and in particular, the effects of this experience not only on your journey to motherhood but life as a whole. Also, the effects of shame. As you know, I made the choice to release Rosa. This wasn't the first time I had been through this experience, however.

I had already chosen to release a baby much earlier on in life, right before I was due to go to London to study for my Master's degree. The man was wrong – very wrong. The timing was wrong, the whole thing was wrong logically. Emotionally, however, it felt right. I loved the fact there was a baby growing. I loved this baby. But I wasn't strong enough to make the choice to change the whole course of my life and, quite frankly, the thought of being tied forever to this perfectly okay, but totally not for me guy was what made me go through with it.

I knew I'd made the right choice, however I refused to allow myself to feel the pain of it, a pain I wouldn't wish on any woman, even though it is the right choice for them and their babies. This shame, the pain, again all held within, which I never spoke about, came back to seriously bite me on the bum when I was ready to become a mum with my husband.

It wasn't with Max – it all started with the first miscarriage. Karma, I thought, for being evil and killing my baby. Yes, those harsh words did spin through my head. How awful we are to ourselves. I've known many women who have had to go through this experience and not once did these words cross my mind for them – only compassion.

And then the second miscarriage. Wow – I really didn't deserve to be a mum. I must be a really, really bad person! So it spiralled until my heart closed and I didn't even realise it. I was going through the motions and being totally normal, having fun and loving my work at the time, and my life was great – except it wasn't. There was nagging doubt, this nagging uncomfortable feeling that I was wrong, I was bad, and I had to be super nice to everyone else just in case they found out how bad I really was.

This is far from an easy story to admit, and I acknowledge at the time of writing this chapter I still have some inner work to do around this as I can still feel a little cringe writing these words. If you're feeling a cringe, write it down, and set the intention of finding out what belief is behind it. I've explored my 'cringe' many times and for me it's all down to not wanting to be visible, sharing of myself as it doesn't feel safe – so nothing to do with the termination at all, and all to do with past life traumas. This is why we can never figure out why we feel what we feel through our minds alone, we have to follow the energy, follow the feeling.

I have faced my dark side enough, however, to feel like I own that part of my life. All the mixed emotions of love, fear, how could I be so stupid to get myself in that position, betrayal, rejection, hurt, frustration at giving away my power and trusting him to take precautions, and sadness. There's a lot to explore, but that is the point, that these experiences push us into delving within and knowing ourselves at a deeper level – and forgiving ourselves for what we didn't know at the time. I own this part of my story enough to talk about it here – it happened and the effects have all converged to bring me here.

I have also explored it on a deeper level for meaning, of which so much opened up because of that experience. This was in terms of the relationship with my mum. We became even closer through this, probably the first time in my adult life I'd been able to ask her for her help. And she was there, as she always was, with unconditional love and support for whatever choice I made. It also meant I was able to understand friends going through this choice and all women who find me and need non-judgemental support, and to understand the deeper meaning of termination.

Whatever your beliefs and feelings on termination right now, the fact is, it happens. It's so important to heal the trauma which follows, hidden or not. It's nearly always the woman who blames herself and is 'blamed' and judged for any choices she makes because of this and carries the physical and emotional pain of this choice, as if the man had absolutely nothing to do with it. We go back to those indoctrinated beliefs around women and sex, women having choice over their decisions and their bodies; women are wrong or bad.

This may have already been done but I wonder sometimes about writing a book turning everything on its head. If men had babies, what would the world look like? Again, let's remember it's not 'men', it's so easy to slip into blame and this does no one any favours. Let's remember it's not men, the gender, but the twisted beliefs and wounds that lead to the distortion in the masculine and feminine energies; the way patriarchy has ruled our way of seeing the world, that sees both genders at its mercy.

Also not taken into account are the baby's role, their views and choices. When I was planning to run an evening healing the effects of termination with two fellow healers, Marina Beech and Olwen Jennings, so much information came flooding through from Rosa, and Olwen's guides too. You read about baby Grace earlier, who came into a situation where her mum made the choice to release her, but actually, that choice meant she was able to move out of an abusive relationship.

The babies I've connected with who are part of this experience have only ever shared love, offered love, and let their mums know there is nothing to forgive. If the mum is ready and wishes to understand the bigger picture behind it, most usually we're shown it. It's likely that there are some baby souls that may be a little more disgruntled. Please don't jump to the automatic assumption this would be your baby and use it to kick yourself with. If you did have this thought, stop right there and see the gift in it – why do you think this may be true? What thought did you have about yourself? Write it down. What if it was true and your baby is disgruntled – but also – what if it wasn't true? Where do you feel the pain of this in your body? Notice everything, it's your path to healing any unresolved trauma. With the many women I've guided to healing around this, I certainly haven't come across any disgruntled baby souls.

This energy did not come through at all in the information we were receiving for our healing evening. One of the key messages to come through was that there was no forgiveness needed because this was part of their soul journey, both theirs and their mum's. By holding onto guilt, you're seeing your baby as a victim – they are very far from this – they are beautiful, powerful souls with choice. There was a real sense that holding onto guilt and finding it hard to forgive yourself kept the babies tied to the experience as well and they were asking for both the mum's and themselves, to be free. Again, no blame, no being unkind to yourself; remember we only know what we know, and then we learn and then we grow.

In terms of your own soul growth, this experience is a biggie, as you'll know already, and Rosa's message below will illuminate this further. Healing through your experience, forgiving yourself, finding and transforming any beliefs that may have arisen from releasing your baby that have led you to believe you're not good enough or don't deserve to be a mum. Finding peace with yourself not only changes how you feel about yourself, it changes your life, physically, energetically and spiritually, and you can play a huge role in healing the collective beliefs which are holding women back.

# The spiritual perspective on termination and shame

I got the sense that in Rosa's message below, she was referring to the female body, but also the body that is earth, and the consciousness she holds. This is the same as us in that we are a body holding our own consciousness. We are all connected to Mother Earth and feel the effects of our treatment of her.

### Rosa on shame

Shame, what is shame? What is this terminology of shame and why is it present in your human form? For it is certainly not an emotion that I feel here where I am now. But this does not help you understand shame and so I will do my best to describe it to you and from whence it came.

Shame is essentially about shame of the body that once gave and gave and gave in its infinite love of the universe and of all beings present in that universe. And it was with no shame that this love was given because this love was for the highest and best of all.

It was a choice to give and a choice to love and a choice to share all of the goodness of the body and all of the life-force energy and all of the beings that could be birthed from it. Yet again, at some point in time, there were many who chose to question this love, this type of love that was all-giving, and all-seeing, and all-knowing of life.

For who were they to not have this love for themselves? Who are they to not have this love and to bottle it up and sell it for all it was worth? Who were they to not have control over this love?

So they took it. They took it for themselves not knowing that they already had it. It was buried so deeply within them they did not realise it. It was the way that they took it that was the instigator and catalyst for the shame that so many of you experience now.

For it was certainly not there before and at some point in time, it will no longer need to be there, present within you. There will be an even deeper understanding of what it is to love and what it means to give and, in particular, give life to another being, whether that be a being born into physical form or a being born back into the loving arms of the whole universe.

## Behind the scenes of termination

So you see, when you ask about the shame that is linked

to a termination, there really is no such thing, because you are not terminating anything or anyone, as no thing and no one can be terminated, and at the very most by a human form, because this is not within your power to terminate and neither is it your choice.

It simply is a birthing of a being into another realm, a realm that may most likely suit that being better at that time than the realm of the earth. When you say you released me, this is exactly what you did – released me from my contract to return to earth in order that I may continue my studies and continue my living from another place – a place where you find me now in the other realms. And yes, including in the baby spirit realm, for I do not always dwell there for I have no notion of yet again returning to your earth, at least not until there comes a point in time when the earth is indeed heaven again.

For this is indeed what the earth was and is – heaven. You simply do not see it that way. It is of your own making that you see it as a hell – a hell on earth – because you choose to remain in the past, choose to remain in those moments of trauma when the world collapsed around you and you did all indeed feel like you were dying.

But, die you did not, and neither have any of your babies, or anyone else's babies. We are simply here moving about the universe, birthed into the realms we are meant to be in right now.

This may well be the realm of the earth or may well be another realm, but know that whatever realm we are in, we are and always will be with you. So do not hold onto the shame that you have killed, or you have terminated, for there are no such words here in the universe. We do not know of this experience of being terminated. We only know of this experience of being birthed.

And as we birth, so too do others birth, as we are continually recycling ourselves into more and more of the experiences we came here for, and it makes no matter to us whether that experience is here with you on earth physically, or here with you in another place or time. We are simply with you, living our lives as we choose to live.

Yet, in your realm, you take these choices as signs of weakness, of something wrong, of something 'bad', of something to admonish and administer pain, either to yourselves or to others whose personal soul journey you do not understand.

It is time to be rid of this shame for it is not a real thing. It has been given to you by others who choose to try and control you and control the choices you make.

They are not ready, nor do they wish you to be ready to see the very real truth of the matter – that matter (form/body/energy) is matter. You cannot make matter come to an end and you cannot make matter, matter, without that matter having a choice in the matter.

I know you often get lost in all my words and this makes me laugh as I am playing with you sometimes when I do this. I know how seriously you can take life and I know how complicated you can make life seem when in reality there are no complications; we simply are.

We are simply here, or we are simply not here. When we are not here with you on earth, we are simply somewhere else, and yet always with you. Do not feel bad from a soul level that you have released your babies. They will always come back to you if that is their want and that is your want and that is part of your plan together.

They feel no pain at the moment of release. They only feel birthed into somewhere else for another adventure until, and if, it is time for them to re-join you in this physical place.

Yet I know that on a human level this is a choice that is far from simple and far from free of pain. But maybe that is the point of this experience for many of you – that you feel this pain, that you are aware of this pain within your physical form. And, yes, also in your soul form – for it is through the experience of this pain and of this shame, and the experience of this loss of your baby, your values, your beliefs of 'thou shalt not kill' your loss of self and who you thought you were.

Because this is what your so-called termination does. It does not terminate your baby soul, for this is not a law of the universe. It terminates, instead, many things about yourself. You can choose to live with this termination of your life as you know it, the termination of yourself as you know it, the termination of how you feel about your own dignity, your values, your sense of self-worth and your own worthiness to be alive in this world.

## A termination of old patterns, beliefs, and controls

This is what a termination is for. And if you are not ready to experience this termination, this death of your old ways, your old patterns and programmes and who you thought yourself to be, then we do not recommend this experience for you.

For you are not ready to go within, so deep within that you often feel you will never come out of it. Never come out of that box of shame that has been programmed into you from almost the beginning of time when others decided that life was there to control, love was there to control, that only 'they' could make your choice of what was right or what was wrong, and not the individual. And most certainly not the woman.

For who was a woman to make a choice of who lives and who dies? Surely it is only the male of the species, the male who himself cannot create life in either your human sense, or universal sense, who must be the one to control, and be in control, of this process of creation.

If it was the woman, then where does that leave the male?

What would happen to the male, to the masculine, to the point of them, if they were not able to control the women? For surely the women would simply give and give and give. What would happen then if we all did just give and give and give?

It is not a concept that can come easily to the male, for there is an energy of take and claim in their being. It is this that has got out of balance. And it is this that must now come full circle and back into balance.

For the female to rise, yes, but for the male to be heard and to be understood and for their fear of being inconsequential, a fear that runs so deep within the veins of the universe, that it affects all things and affects all life.

Once the male is recognised and honoured as a master creator in their own right, once they are recognised as the being that must be visible within the process of creation, that creation is indeed the balance of both the male and the female. Then it is that a true creation can happen.

The creation of life on all planets as and when an individual soul so chooses to incarnate, or so chooses to be birthed. Or chooses to experience the depths of the pain of loss in order to heal and to lift and to rise through this pain and understand that they are not only living this pain now, but indeed playing out an ancient, ancient story of fear – fear of the wiping out of the masculine.

And it is to this fear that we must now all turn to ease and to coddle the male in order for the world to feel a safe place once more. A safe place to be. A safe place without fear or without shame. For in reality there cannot be any such thing.

And so we honour you women who have made this choice. Made this choice to destroy a life before it had even begun, for you have destroyed nothing and no one but the fear and the shame within yourselves.

And so this too is a service, a service of giving and a service of love. We honour you for this. It is with our love and blessing that soon this will no longer be a need to perform. That this will no longer be a deed that needs to be seen or taken. For there will be no thing that needs to be terminated – for all there will be – is love.

And so it is.

Our infinite blessings,

Rosa

This message blew my mind, as most of them do. Take your time with them, these are huge concepts to get your head around as they knock into all sorts of programmed and unconscious beliefs and judgements we may hold, myself included, about termination. What I've learnt through channelling Rosa is that the answers I expect to hear are nowhere near what she tells me. As you can see, there is always a much, much bigger picture than what we physically can see or know. We can only do what is right for us in each moment and do our best to find resolution to our decisions, our traumas, and find peace with ourselves through our physical minds and bodies as well as discovering the deeper meaning of them. We can of course find out if we choose to.

Her message highlights again where the masculine energy and patriarchy feel they have a right of control over women's choices, their bodies, and creation. All driven from fear. But why, even now, is it most often male judges and politicians who feel they have control over what is or isn't right, using 'God rules' as a reason? Where did this belief come from, is it true for you? And where is the responsibility of the male here? It takes two to create: egg and sperm. To stay out of blame it's important to remember that although these are conscious decisions on what they feel is right or wrong, it's coming from an unconscious place and energy. We'll be looking more at this in Part 2 of the book. For now, feel into your own truth and right of choice as a sovereign being. Knowing your baby also has and had choice as a sovereign being. The behind the scenes picture is huge.

Receiving support in healing and understanding the why of this experience is so important. With me, it kept me in hiding, not wanting to be visible for fear of being 'found out'. This was in all aspects of work and relationships. As mentioned before, your journey to motherhood is not a separate aspect of your life; your life is one, whole, journey, all calling you back to the truth of who you are.

## Life and death

There was one line in Rosa's message that drew my attention one time I was re-reading it. The sentence when she spoke about termination being the death of your old ways, your old patterns and programmes and who you thought yourself to be. Being in the situation where you have this choice to make helps you face long-held collective beliefs about sexual authority over your body, your power as a sovereign being to have the right to choose. It also made me want to understand more about death being a part of life and what unconscious beliefs I was holding that makes me shy away from the word and dread the experience, not of my own death but other people, particularly my loved ones. I realised this fear came from unresolved trauma around the losses I'd experienced.

I also remembered Rosa's words in her earlier message about the New Earth, that 'they', whoever they are, made death bad. I presume before whatever traumatic event occurred for us to feel such fear and confusion, death was viewed in a very different way. By fearing death we hold ourselves back from truly living.

As humans we are far more fearful of public speaking than of death – the fear of judgement, really. But certainly fear of death is right up there. I have experienced many losses – grandparents, my mum and dad, friends, pets, and, of course, five beautiful baby souls.

And even though I know what I know, even though I do what I do working between the worlds of life and death and many different realms, and absolutely knowing that there is no such thing as death, but a rebirthing into another realm, it still doesn't take away the fact it hurts like nothing else. The human side of loss is one of our greatest challenges and lessons. It can diminish or you can grow from it. It is your choice. Grief cracks you wide open and how you navigate it is such a personal journey.

In recent Soul Plan Readings with clients, when I've accessed their life before life or in between life stage, twice I've found myself watching my client having a conversation with 'death', or the grim reaper, whatever name you put to it. One of them was having afternoon tea with this energy! The insight myself and my clients gained from this was that we hold such fear of death and a skewed sense of what it actually is. We've been trained to fear it as the worst imaginable event. What's behind this fear – as with everything – is whether our beliefs around dying are working for our benefit and good, or as a way of keeping us in fear, less adventurous and more controlled.

How myself and my clients felt this energy of 'death' was one of compassion and teaching, a guide helping them to review their life and, if it was time, to step into something new. The something new was to pass into the realm of spirit for one of my clients – and for my other client, it was to step into the body of a baby soul and come to earth again. So death is really an opportunity for something new, a new beginning, a new vibration and experience when you're ready to learn something new – leave one place and into another. It may take a while for our human selves to catch up with this concept and that's okay, we're all heading in our way through to new realities.

We've read a message about baby loss in Chapter 1 of this book. The message below from Source/Creator/God – whatever term you describe unconditional love of all that is – concerns death itself. The energy of the word is enough to dip even the lightest energy. So I truly hope this message offers some healing and understanding from the spiritual perspective.

**Source on the illumination of death**

> Death, the very word carries such a low energy and makes us feel miserable. How about instead we talk about death

as illumination? Illumination into the light of all that is. Illuminating the love we felt and continue to feel.

Death is but a whisper of the light that shows us that life goes on, that nothing truly dies but simply changes form.

Death is the acknowledgment of a life well-lived, that they can now return home, satisfied that their mission is complete for now.

Death is a word, a mere word, that conjures up thoughts and feelings and emotions of loss and pain. However, it is only a word. A word that spells doom and destruction. Is there another word for you, that will lift you more during this time of need?

See it as a passing, a phase, a transition, an acknowledgement of a life well-lived and well-loved and well-learnt. Can there be another word now there is a knowing that nothing and no one truly ever dies? Could this word be illumination? Illuminating all we felt and feel in order to grow from it, to connect more deeply with ourselves and our lost loved ones? To illuminate love?

## How spirit view death

Life and death in your world are seen very differently from ours. All there is, is transition from one plane to another and, as we rise up through the planes, we know we have achieved ever greater mastery of ourselves and are in closer contact to our God-self than ever before.

This is a beautiful thing as we leave the ones on our current plane to travel ever higher, for there are always opportunities and chances to re-meet our souls here, whether in this lifetime or the next. We always rejoice when these souls are seen to lift themselves higher and even higher to re-join us on our own planes, until it is time yet again for our own selves to be lifted higher and our own selves to be joined with the ever-increasing higher beings of light.

Do you see that this notion of death to us is not a notion at all but merely an opportunity for us to go even higher into the light, the light of who we truly are at our very essence and core.

The core of who we are is the pureness of this light and the game of life and the game of death is to swirl ever upwards towards that light, expanding, growing, and forever changing in our form and level of 'beingness' until we too simply disappear into the light and become one with all that is.

This is our game, little ones, so do not take this life of yours so seriously, as all you are doing is resisting this urge to return to the light. Understand instead that the light is coming, the light is all around you, and that you are already the light. It just so happens that you are on a plane of existence where that light is heavier and therefore cannot be seen or felt so clearly.

Its visibility is hidden, often beneath clouds of energy that have no place in your world. Can you see that by choosing to return to this earth plane, and live on this particular plane of existence, you have chosen to lighten this energy with your presence? It is these darker clouds of energy that disappear and not the light energy that is you.

It is time, our little ones, to transcend this darker energy once and for all and we are helping you with this right now. To transcend the all and everything of this particular energy that resides on your planet that has no right to be there, as this is in fact the energy of death on your planet.

The death of your spirit, of hope, the death of your loved ones in a ball of fire and a ball of gloom. The despondency as you feel you can no longer hold the light on this planet and therefore it may be best to retreat and leave them to it.

However, this is not what you came onto this planet to do. The exhaustion that you feel about the world and its people.

The greed, loathing, and the legacies of hatred that continue to bounce back and forth between the generations, are the precise reasons that you have chosen to be here, in the here and now. It's time to put an end to the shame and the blame and the killings based on fear of lack and not of love. Through the knowing of the light you are.

It is through your healing and shining your light, the light of your babies and future babies that are lifting these darker energies back into love too. There is no circumnavigating the pain of loss and no words that can make loss any easier, feeling it is currently a part of life. It is a great teacher of self. This is the same whether we feel we have lost who we thought we were or what our life was about, or the loss of another. We have to be with the emotions that come from loss, they have not come out of the blue because of it, they were already there. When you allow yourself to see them, it eases the need to kick yourself about what you did or didn't do, or if you're weak or strong, or stay in the suffering.

Knowing there is no such thing as dying but a transformation, knowing your babies and loved ones are experiencing their own 'death' as joy as they move back into wholeness to wherever they need to be right now, knowing you haven't 'lost' them or yourself because they are no longer here physically, is a deep and painful journey. At some point in time, when you're ready, you'll begin to feel the light of you again, the you that is the same but different. The you that has grown through this experience.

## What's the point of it all? What are the benefits? Where is it taking us?

I asked Rosa, where is all this taking us? The benefits to the individual are clear and the rewards of our own courage to look deeper within are truly infinite. These rewards, however, are not only for your benefit, but also for that of your children and future children. Because the less heartache and pain there is, and the more we become aware of and meet our own needs, the more free our children become. Not least because they'll have less traumatised and stressed parents but more aware parents who recognise that their children are not here to fill them up and give them what they lack, but to fill up their own selves; that each and every individual has their own plan and mission and is a perfect piece of a beautiful and infinite puzzle.

As parents we are here to guide our children as best we can onto their own path – and not a path we think they should be on. Our traumas and conditioning are passed on through generation after generation. What a beautiful gift for your future child to have freed your own self from any or as much pain as possible, or even the intention and awareness of doing so before they even arrive, so they don't have to carry it along the line.

The children of the New Earth, which is covered in the next part of this book, are coming to change the way the world operates to one of cooperation and connection and not competition and disconnection. They are coming to move the world further away from the effects of patriarchy and separation and bring more balance. This includes in areas such as education, medicine, religion, politics, and business, and bringing new insights and new solutions so that humans, Mother Earth and life on earth, can thrive to their best and infinite potential.

Rosa's message below shows us what is possible and where we are heading if we choose to. Everything is energy. Feel into the energy now of happiness, then feel into the energy of sadness. We are not our emotions; they are signposts to where we're at. There's a well-known saying that what you see on the outside is what is going on inside. And what you are projecting out from the inside, you will see on the outside. If you view and feel life through a more joyful lens, you will see more joyful things and draw more joyful experiences to you. The same is true if you see the world as a dangerous place or a place of lack. Your mind will look for evidence of it, and your energy will match the energy of danger or lack and manifest it. Rosa describes these as fields of consciousness and asks us to look at which fields we are wishing to play in.

Rosa offers a view of a potential future.

## The final word, for now, from Rosa

Look, my darling, look at the sight of heaven here on earth. Can you see it? Can you feel it? Can you feel the wonder of what it will be like when all children feel free to roam and play, to live and to explore in this playground of life?

To find their own way and their own path of freedom, and not at the behest of their parents, but at the behest of their own souls; their own souls who wish to fly free and to love and to play and to explore as the geniuses they are and not the geniuses that their parents and others see them as through their own limited eyes.

Imagine a life without limit. Imagine a life without the need to do or say or to be like everyone else in order to feel worthy, in order to feel loved, in order to feel they belong, are a part of. Because of course everyone is a part of and yet separate from the source of all the light from which they came.

You will see yourselves as souls of light, lighting up the path ahead for your children, and your children's children, to be free of all the patterning and conditioning from those dark times of the past. Those dark times when you were not allowed to fly and be free.

The many of you who do not see this yet will be abhorred and will struggle with this concept of freedom, and this concept of every soul being a whole and equal part of the whole. The only reason is that you have been trained to know yourselves as better, trained to be better, to be more than; enriched with the DNA of the souls who did not want to see this freedom of the love of earth but instead wanted to take, and stop, and control this love of the earth for it is something you would not and perhaps will never be able to fully comprehend in your minds.

And this is fine. This is not a bad thing for we will still need the darkness in which we can shine our light. It is just that the light will be able to shine ever more brightly out into the darkness now, once many more of us have switched on these lights.

So, do not fear if you feel you are the one with the darkness lying inside, for you too are playing a fine role in this New Earth. And if this role is your choice and you are enjoying this choice, then please do go ahead and choose it, for you are no less valued for it.

Yet if you no longer wish to play the role of the malevolent benefactor, then maybe it is time to think again of the choices that you have made and are making each and every day in the playing out of this role. For the truth is, is it making you happy? Are you a happy soul with happy thoughts or are you a dark soul with darker thoughts?

And if you are, again this is fine, for there is much to learn from the darkness, and we welcome you for it. However, if it is a case of you coming out of that darkness and trying on the coat of light for a while, we are grateful and honour you for it.

## Soul journey

Do you see that it is in every soul's progression from the dark into the light, and back again, that we can all learn and adjust and play in the fields of all consciousness that are out there? It is entirely dependent on us as to which fields we play in. We may wish to play in the happy field for a short time, or maybe you wish to play in the grumpy field for a short time – and all is fine and all is welcome. For do you not see that you are all and everything of the all and everything? Therefore it is your absolute own choice as to which field you wish to choose at any particular moment of time.

You may see that at some point in time you enjoy one particular field over another and you will begin to step more and more into that field as the other fields become a more distant memory.

Perhaps you will feel nostalgia as you look back at the fun times you spent in the darker fields of consciousness, playing and trying on the clothes that didn't fit you so well, in order to send you jumping into another set of clothes – until you realise that you have no clothes at all other than the ones you choose to dress in.

What of the fields of consciousness in which these new children will play? Will they be playing in the darker sides of the field that you are willing to show them? Perhaps even intentionally showing them in order to create a harm that they then have to work their way out of, much as you may have done, or are doing, in order to find a happier field of play?

Or do you wish for these new children to merely have a knowing, a nostalgia and, yes, even perhaps dip their toe into the darker energies of the fields of consciousness in order to feel the gratitude of no longer having to remain there for as long as is necessary to learn the very quick lesson of remembrance of the past in order to build on it for a new future?

## What life do you wish for your children?

Which future do you see for your child? A lighter, brighter future of play and of understanding? A lighter, brighter future of playing with the concept of the dark and yet in full knowing that this is not their path and that they are indeed the next path out of it? Or would you like to see them being dragged continuously down into the dark and the mire that has plagued your world for so many eons of time?

And if so, why? If this is because you cannot find your way out, then  so be it. You will and can be helped to jump into other timelines of happiness and joy. And if it is not your choice, for you choose not to be the person who is able to let go of the past hurts and resentment of lifetimes of learning, then so be it. For it is your choice, and the little ones who come to you are to be our bravest soldiers who are once again prepared to step in and show the possibility of another way, another life, another time where you were not this.

This is not a case of one being more than the other; simply a case of two halves being shown in order to bring about the light, the opportunity for the light to be shone within, both as a way of balance and healing that has never yet been seen before.

Our light-warriors and our lightworkers are here to assist both yourselves and your children in this balancing of the light and this understanding of the dark – for surely they are one and the same thing. Some do truly believe the dark to be light, and some do truly see the light to be the dark, and this is what we are turning our attention to now.

All light and all dark are one and the same thing. The only difference lies in the fields of consciousness in which you find yourself and where you play, which will determine the reality of what you are seeing, experiencing, and witnessing. And we would like you to see both the dark in the light and the light in the dark, for this is the truth of all of life.

Yet by doing so, there cannot be any dark, for all is therefore of the light and all is therefore bringing the light. Do you see this, my dear? The fields in which you choose to play determine the fit and the balance of the light within the dark, and the dark within the light. Surely it is time for you all to see that without the light, or the dark, there is only a return to nothingness.

## The All of nothingness

A return to the nothingness of all there ever was before. It is this fear of nothing, this being nothing, that reduces you all to play with the concept of light and dark. And yet what is so terrifying about the nothingness? For it is in the nothingness that we are all in abundance. We are all in this nothingness together as one huge whole of the whole of all-ness. The all-ness of the all and everything.

There is, in fact, nothing to fear of the nothing. The no-thing. For you never were and never have been and never will be anything other than no-thing. For a thing cannot possibly be anything other than separate and a thing can never be anything other than apart. And so if we are no-thing, then we are indeed all whole.

And this, my dear, is the secret of the universe for you to reveal to the masses. And it is in the whole souls of the children, who are coming onto your planet now, who will show you that they are indeed nothing, for they are indeed everything.

And so it is.

As we draw to a close on Part 1 of this book, all you have read so far may well be all you need to know for now. Your own individual experience may be enough to explore, heal through, and know the beautiful gift this also brings to your children and future children. If you are on a challenging journey to motherhood I know it's hard to think of anything else other than what's going on for you. So head straight to the conclusion of this book to feel a sense of completion. Sit quietly with yourself, meditate or journal on what you've already read and be in awe of yourself. Feel the inklings of curiosity and possibility as you allow Rosa's words to soak into your consciousness – you are the miracle; you are a creator. You are a woman who is powerful enough to welcome, hold and birth a new soul. You are love, you are loved, you are enough.

As Rosa shared during one of my livestream meditations one day:

Hold onto you

Hold onto love

Hold onto the miracle

You are the miracle.


For those of you who are curious and perhaps further along your self-healing or spiritual development then read on. Or perhaps you are a spiritual teacher, guide or mentor, either knowingly or unknowingly for the moment, here to support these children of the light and their parents; here to play your role in healing the mother wound and bring balance between the masculine and the feminine. The next few chapters will look at why the energy of creation has become so out of balance; how your own individual healing has an effect on many more people than you and your children; how it plays a role in healing and lifting the earth and, ultimately, the universe. Yes, you really are that powerful!

In Part 2 we'll be looking at the collective, how you are a beautiful, precious piece of an enormous puzzle. We'll be going deeper into who you are and the story you're playing out; deeper into the energies of the Divine masculine, Divine feminine, and the Divine Child. Who and what are they? Where we are seeing the imbalance in our lives and where, how, and why the feminine has been suppressed, as well as the role of the Church.

Through this lens, Rosa guides us to looks at reasons why people experience infertility; how these energies have been corrupted and how we can bring them back into balance, and bring ourselves back into balance through finding our power and connecting to our sense of self. This next part of the book also looks at the driving energy behind infertility and medical interventions such as IVF, how as women we've given our power away, and how we are all moving towards a sense of self-belief and self-love – valued, heard, and safe to express our unique voice out into the world.

# Part TWO

# Chapter 11
## Healing the Divine Feminine, the Divine Masculine and Meeting the Divine Child

What is the Divine Feminine and why is everyone in spiritual circles talking about it? There's been a sense of real, more widespread change since 2012, when there was a huge energy shift in the world. But it was in 2017, when women began speaking out about abuse by producer Harvey Weinstein and other men in corporate media, that saw women speak out more, command more and rise into their power, as well as an awareness of this powerful energy in the world.

The goings-on in Hollywood did throw me slightly. Not because I found the revelations unexpected, or surprising, but because for many women and young girls, including myself as a teenager and young woman, sexual manipulation has been accepted as something that happens and you get on with it. Quite frankly – wtf! How did so many of us ever just accept this as a way of being and get on with it?

For me, this news story was a very real representation of the tide turning, of women waking up to their power. Not power over men or other women, or anyone or anything, in fact, but in their knowingness and empowerment, feeling secure in who they are. Having a right to their voice.

Bearing in mind that we all hold both male and female energies, and therefore this isn't about gender, the message that came through from Source at the time is this:

> The happenings in Hollywood are a profound statement to the world that female energy will no longer accept its disempowerment. It is time for balance and unity and this can't take place until both males and females see themselves as equals, with equal respect, equal priority, and equal right to live their lives as they choose.

> See this as a start on the physical plane of what more is to

come as energies become more balanced and people begin to see the light they hold within themselves and the light of each other. There will come a time when living without this balance will be impossible and an ancient relic of the past.

It is indeed the time and the earth is shifting to allow this to happen.

The result of these allegations, starting with the media focusing on one courageous woman, although there are thousands who came before her over the generations, saw the beginning of the Me Too campaign – an opportunity for women to speak about their experiences of sexual harassment and worse.

The sexual abuse scandals in churches and in children's homes and at the BBC and in sport and ever, wider areas of life – all of this pain courageously faced by those, both women and men, who took the lead and spoke of their experiences, this, in turn, helped others to speak about their pain, their abuse. It's horrific to see, but unless we do, it can't change. It may help to think of these issues as a deeply wounded energy that requires healing, rather than any personality involved. Take responsibility for how you feel when reading this particular section, journal, allow the feelings, practise EFT tapping to keep you in your centre. EFT, emotional freedom technique, is a very simple and powerful energy healing tool, a bit like acupuncture but without the needles. You gently tap on various end points of your meridian lines and it is one of the best tools I know to reduce anxious feelings and stress, fearful memories and much more. Through tapping you are calming down your flight, fight, freeze response. It's definitely worth looking up.

This suppression and the energy, trait or need to have 'power over' someone else, has been going on for eons. To bring it home to you, this energy is an easy one to slip into with our children. We would rarely shout at someone else for some perceived minor behavioural slip, so why is it viewed as acceptable or normal to shout at a child? Is it because they have less power? Maybe you were shouted at as a child, how did this make you feel? A wound is a wound and we're all playing this abuse of power energy out in our lives somewhere, slipping between the power over someone to being disempowered. There's no blame here, see it as an energy that needs love and healing so it can transform into true power – which I believe is the peaceful power that comes with self-belief.

One of the reasons for this energy being so prevalent across the world, as Rosa says in her message on shame, is the deep-seated fear, held by the imbalanced masculine energy, that men are actually inconsequential to creation. They fear the 'mother', creation energy. The masculine is obviously so necessary for creation but this fear of being inconsequential to life is unconscious, deeply buried and carried through generation upon generation and not seen or known. Just played out in various ways of controlling women. I can see how this belief became so out of balance and that the only way men/the masculine energy knew how to be meaningful was to control those who create – women and Mother Earth herself.

## We're all re-enacting the ancient stories of the suppression of the feminine

I am no theologian but, in my perception, you only have to turn to the Bible to see the obvious patriarchy and control in existence over two thousand years ago – and it was happening long before that. The story of Adam and Eve highlights how the energies of masculine and feminine have been made conscious by turning them into form – into two separate people in order to help our human minds make these intangible energies something we can more easily understand. Was Eve (representing the feminine energy) really the cause of sin, as has been written? This is buried deeply in the psyche of women, that somehow women are wrong, have done something wrong and we have to make up for this mistake, this desire and temptation. It's also buried deep in the psyche of men, which is why it's so important for men to feel comfortable with looking at their own healing journey.

The story of the Red Tent cites the story of Dinah, daughter of Jacob, who was father to twelve sons, including Joseph of the technicolour dream coat fame. But the story is all about Jacob and his sons.

Where was Dinah? Her story of forgiveness is so powerful. Mary Magdalene's story was hidden too. She was vilified as a prostitute when in truth she was the equal to Christ in all of her healing and mastery of self, Christ's partner in every sense from what has been channelled in books such as Anna, Grandmother of Jesus and also researched by theologians such as Dr Karen King and Meggan Watterson. I highly recommend Meggan Watterson's book, Mary Magdalene Revealed, to give you another perspective on this story, as well as Claire Heartsong's, Anna, Grandmother of Jesus.

I often work with the energy of Lilith: in our human way of looking at life, the first woman to be banished from the Garden of Eden by Adam for refusing to lie beneath him and be subservient, or so the story goes. Lilith is often portrayed as the serpent that tempted Eve with the apple that brought the downfall of man. She has been vilified – along with snakes – ever since this story took hold. Snakes with their connection to the earth and the kundalini energy and the Divine Feminine have frightened the masculine energy so much; Mother Mary has been depicted as standing on a serpent – literally standing on her own sexuality and power, squashing it or rising above it as if it was separate from her. More pressure piled on women to do the same and live up to the 'image' of Mother Mary as portrayed by some.

Saint Patrick is famous and celebrated for banishing all the snakes from Ireland. The snakes perhaps representing the Divine Feminine? Ireland was home to ancient Celtic Druids, referred to as philosophers, who believe in the immortality of the soul and reincarnation.

Druids then and now live in an equal society with men and women having equal authority. Like many indigenous cultures across the world, druids honour nature and humankind, live in harmony with nature, respect the seasons, the ancestors and nature spirits.

This way of life and shift in philosophy occurred gradually. I don't want to vilify Saint Patrick, a man who was the forerunner to Roman Catholicism in pagan Ireland in the 5th century, who likely just wanted to spread the word of God as he saw it, speak his own truth, with love. However, he's been caught up in this tale somehow. It was around the 8th century when the pope appointed the first "inquisitors of heretical depravity", that saw an end to druidic practises in Ireland. Others were sent to places like Iona in Scotland to tame the female druid priestesses. Rome had such a need for control and obedience: this was the beginning of burning witches and disempowering women and those who didn't follow the Roman Catholic Church's rules and beliefs. A regime ruled through fear. Livescience.com mentions a line in an 8th-century hymn that sums up the attitude of the day that asks for God's protection from the spells of women, blacksmiths, and druids.

Why was there such terror around women and their ability to create, and a need to suppress any practices that celebrated Mother Earth, to the point of burning, humiliating, disempowering and controlling them? It is through this power and these gifts we are being offered the opportunity to reclaim our natural gifts. To be proud of our connection and miracle creating abilities and to use them for the greater good to birth and create, instead of feeling ashamed, humiliated, and wrong for being able to bring about such life-enriching magic.

The misrepresentation that Lilith was trying to bring down Eve can be perceived differently. She tempted Eve to show her there was another way; that she didn't need to be subservient to Adam, that they were in fact equals. In whatever way this story goes, it is one that helps our conscious minds understand the intangible energies at play and the imbalance between the masculine and the feminine.

## A cultural example of the suppression of the feminine

Saint Patrick has popped up in my writing for some reason, maybe he's calling for someone to channel his story? But he's here, so I'll continue with Ireland as a representation of how the feminine has been disempowered. Ireland is the most magical land with so much history and power. I have many friends and clients there and also run retreats within the pyramids of Ard Na Ri. I've been shown two past lives where I lived in Ireland and I feel a strong pull there. It is stunningly beautiful, welcoming and alive with life and mystery, yet the abuse and control of women and children, the control over women's bodies and choices, stains the land and the energetic well-being of women and men. As I said, I'm no theologian but maybe the story of Saint Patrick is really a metaphor about the Divine Feminine being driven out, beaten out even of this hugely powerful land?

It was only in 1965 that Ireland dropped the practice of 'churching'. Churching is thought to derive from a Jewish purification rite, where the sin of childbirth was washed away. It's mentioned in the Bible that Mary was 'purified' after giving birth. Churching in Ireland was when the new mum was given a blessing by the male priest and gratitude for the safe arrival of their baby – but only if she were married and nicely presented. Underlying the practice was a cleansing; much like menstruation, childbirth made a woman unholy or unclean. Churching allowed the 'unclean' women to re-enter the church in a state of grace. Women were viewed as unclean because birth resulted from sexual activity – sexual abstinence and virginity being viewed as holy.

How did this twisted sense of creation and birthing new life become so ingrained and accepted so powerfully that we see the effects continue to play out in daily lives, in views around sex, and in particular women and sex?

Former president of Ireland, Professor Mary McAleese, speaking at a conference – Women the Vatican Couldn't Silence – in 2019, quoted from a book of theology, Love and Responsibility, by the late Pope St John Paul II. It states that in an act of sex in marriage, the woman is "a comparatively passive partner whose function is to accept and experience. For the purpose of the sexual act it is enough for her to be passive and unresisting, so much so that it can even take place without her volition while she is in a state in which she has no awareness at all of what is happening – for instance when she is asleep or unconscious."

While Pope John Paul became a Saint, male theologians and priests, such as Father Sean Fagan who questioned Pope John Paul, were silenced. Such deeply held beliefs and so much trauma resulting from them in all walks of life, not just within the Catholic Church but other religions, many systems, institutions and cultures. It's really time to question everything we have been told, by whom and why, and find your own truth about who you are, what feels right or not for you. These are the changing times as we all awake to what has been hidden within.

Remember to be aware of any blame or victim energy that we're all moving beyond as best we can in these changing times. Blame, judgement, victimhood, this is not who you are – it's an energy. Everyone, no matter what their beliefs, what side of the fence they sit on, is doing the best they can with what they know at the time. And then we grow, and then we rise until hopefully one day we'll rarely be feeling them at all.

You absolutely have the power and ability to approach all of this from a place of curiosity and empowerment. I asked Rosa about the sexual energy and how sex is seen from a higher perspective.

**Rosa talks about the energy of lust**

Take this energy of lust as an example of how you have been told it is a 'wrong' thing, a 'bad' thing, a 'woman' thing even as it is the woman who has often been seen to incite lust in another.

However, is this the truth? For it is certainly not our truth as we sit and watch it from here. For there is no greater energy driving us forward than lust. It is lust that allows us to throw caution to the winds. It is lust that kicks us out of our patterns and behaviours that have so often kept us hidden and quiet.

It is lust that can drive us and motivate us to create and explore and live life as we never have experienced before. Do you see now why this energy of lust has been dubbed a 'bad' thing? That this energy of lust has been marked as the energy of all sinners and those sinned upon? Do you understand why this lustful energy of life and joy has been deemed to be so dangerous it must be controlled at all costs?

And usually at the cost of the human life, human love and human privation? Because it is an energy that can rise up out of nowhere and demand its pleasure. Can you see why they do not wish you to have this pleasure? Can you see why they do not wish you to run free with this energy? Is it perhaps because they want to hold onto it all for themselves? To take it and harness it and use it for their ends and not for the greater good of anyone other than themselves?

For this is a twisted lust, just as there is a twisted love. A twisted love that has held people small and under the cosh of another for fear of them being alone. And much like this, so too has this energy of lust been corrupted to meet the ends of the few and not the needs of the masses.

The need to be free, to express, to explore, to master this lust – that was once such a 'good' thing to be seen to have. This lust for life and procreation and creation, for this is what lust is. It is the energy of life. It has just been twisted and distorted into the one thing where this lust has left someone feeling they have power over another. That it is okay for one to have but not another.

And this is what is wrong in your society. That a whole half of your population have been cut off from their ability to feel lust because they have been told over very many generations that lust is evil, lust is bad, lust is something that men have and can so often 'get you into trouble'.

That it is not the men who can 'get you into trouble' but the lust that you are not allowed to have but which you can incite in men – that is the trouble.

This is the wrong thing. This is the misinterpretation of this energy that has been carried through for many years after many years. Do you now see why this energy was one that the men chose to suppress? Because they wished to suppress you, the very life force that was you, the life force of lust that is the force of abundance and creation – for they wished to take this all for themselves.

But they have not done a great job, for it has not served either the male or the female. For the balance has tipped from one of lust for life and joy and abundance to one of lust for greed and pain and control.

No one can be blamed for it is surely the case that if energy is not allowed to flow, then it will not flow. It will become stuck and distorted and transformed into something other than it was. And so, my dears, it is time to look at your own sense of lust. For your teenagers certainly have it and this is not to be seen as an embarrassing thing; it is only to be seen as a lesson in having and accessing and celebrating this energy – not for the love of lust but for the love of life this lust gives.

For that lust to be harnessed within the self as the life force it is, not to take from others or demand from others but to recognise as a compatible energy in which you give and receive of life itself.

This is not 'giving away your sex'. This is very much not the same as giving anything of yourself away that you do not wish to give. This lust is the powerful force that enables you to live your life from your place of power, from your place of saying no, until you meet it in another to be shared and boosted and exerted out into the universe as an energy of life force, of pleasure, of joy, of fun and of love, always of love.

Love for self, love for another with whom you wish to share and experience this powerful form of lust. Lust from a place of loving.

Rosa's message above spells out clearly that lust, which may be a sexual lust, is a life-force energy, a life-giving energy, a creative energy. One that is sacred and not about giving away or taking from, but owning and being in from a place of love. Harnessing your own life force energy for good. We'll read on in the chapters below why the masculine wished to demonise it and make it a 'bad' thing for women to feel.

How about now you set the intention of feeling the energy of lust. Play with it, see what happens. Notice what thoughts come up, how your body reacts. Ask to have the highest truth and understanding of lust. Lust is life, turn off the programming that tells you otherwise and enjoy the sovereign power of it.

## Dark history coming to light

More and more of Ireland's dark history is coming to light. I have my own connection to the Tuam babies. Tuam is a town in County Galway in Ireland. This was an extremely dark episode in the Church's history when a vault, a former septic tank at a Catholic home where unmarried mothers were sent to give birth between 1925 and 1961, was discovered to be filled with the bodies of a currently estimated 800 babies and young children.

This horror was revealed during excavations in 2016. I knew I would visit Tuam one day after going on retreat with my now tribe of magnificent women healers, when I discovered I was able to release the stuck or trauma energy of babies and other souls from the earth at another former mum and baby home in Ireland. I'd always put off going there, it felt too big and too dark. On one of my trips to Ireland however, to run a retreat, my friend Hilary wasn't able to pick me up and so I took the bus. I didn't know this but the bus stopped in Tuam. All it took was a 10 minute stop in the town to activate the most massive healing I have ever experienced and one that was clearly in my soul contract.

I have been torn as to whether to share this story because of the unimaginable trauma being lived by those whose babies or relatives of the mums involved. However, I've been reassured by Irish friends and my guides that revealing this will help bring much-needed healing. There is no hiding anymore for these babies. As with all trauma, it has to be seen in as gentle and loving a manner as possible before it can be moved through.

When I returned home from Ireland I was feeling all sorts of crazy, like I'd been taken over by grief, anger, resentment, sadness and much more. I knew it wasn't mine. I had a session booked with one of my mentors, the incredible Sharon Brown, who also happens to be Irish. As soon as I told her what was going on and she tuned in, she asked, "Have you been to Tuam?" She didn't even know I'd been in Ireland that weekend.

But all she could see was hundreds of souls in my energy field and her guides showed her Tuam. This is the miracle and magic of being connected; we have access to all sorts of knowledge and information. Over the next two hours, we proceeded to call all these souls forward and up and out of where aspects of their soul energy had been trapped. Some were just happy to go straight to the light, some needed healing, some were very vocal in how they felt, some were extremely angry. And others declared they were coming straight back to change the way institutions are run, not for revenge but because they want to bring in a new way and ensure this lack of humanity never happens again. It was a profound moment for both myself and Sharon to be part of this freeing up for these souls, but also the land and this dark energy that had been stuck there.

There is much more to this story and not a lot has happened so far in an official capacity to honour these souls and their families or bring about justice. I truly hope, knowing that these little ones are now at peace, that change is coming and will bring healing and resolution.

Revealing dark moments, such as Tuam, has been brutal for so many to face, but ultimately also healing. Awful experiences can be kept hidden; even if seen clearly, they can remain hidden because no one wants to face them and call them out. Control through the use of shame and humiliation is a powerful tool; it keeps things hidden and piles pressure on individuals to stay safe within societal norms, to not stand up  and speak out. This leads only to silent, personal questioning and most likely suffering, rather than calling them out and rocking the boat.

When issues are no longer hidden, painful as it is at the time, the process of acceptance and healing can begin, life transforms. In 2019 there was a change in the law concerning abortion in Ireland, meaning that women and medical staff were no longer at risk of being prosecuted for making this choice or supporting women in making this choice. This was a huge turnaround in one aspect of women reclaiming themselves and their right to choose.

My wish is that those women who had to endure secret terminations or being sent away to mother and baby homes or forced to give up their babies, are supported through their trauma. I'm not singling out Ireland; it's simply one example I know about and which is close to my heart. For sure, the extreme nature of this abuse against the feminine and the creation process goes on elsewhere. But why? Why has the feminine been so brutalised and disempowered?

## What's all of this got to do with me you may ask?

You may be wondering what this has to do with your own journey to motherhood. The answer is that underneath the stories, underneath your story and your journey and the emotions that are brought up because of it, is the most ancient story of all, that of creation and our evolution as humans in a spiritual context. We all carry the wounds of the past, deeply embedded in our psyche, and played out across millennia in various different guises, by many different actors. You are one of these actors now, playing out this ancient story in order to restore balance, in order to create in balance, whether that is a new life, or your own way of living.

One incredible woman who came to me for support on her journey to motherhood was experiencing the physical pain of this ancient story and also this lifetime pain around her own birth in the form of endometriosis. There's a whole science on metaphysical health to explore if you are interested. In Lise Bourbeau's book, Your Body's Telling You: Love Yourself!, she suggests that endometriosis may stem from a fear of bearing children and the possible consequences of childbirth. This can come from a woman's own mother and often from past lives. This fear and anticipated pain causes confusion in a woman's reproductive organs. On a spiritual level, you have a strong desire for a child, strong enough that your body responds by creating an extra uterus as the tissue from the lining of the uterus (the endometrium) back up into the pelvis and fallopian tubes. This tissue adheres to organs and/or the pelvic wall and continues to function as uterine tissue. Intense fear of the implications of childbirth is, however, holding all the cards.

The healing journeys myself and my client went on travelled way back into the past to reveal the insights of her wounded feminine aspect. In one session, Mary Magdalene came through to pass this message below onto her, which she has allowed me to share.

> We will no longer live under a cloak of sadness, we will no longer live under a cloak of shame at our pain. We will reveal and celebrate our pain and live in our pain, until that pain no longer needs to be revealed. We can lift this pain from the shoulders of all women. This is the soul of a long line of many women who are here to say no more to the pain. No more to the shame and the hiding of that pain. For that pain is real and once it is acknowledged as such it no longer has to be, or it can no longer be.

> Know this soul is now released from this pain and it is now she must set out on her work to release the pain of others and to lift the shroud of secrecy and the cloak of damage that has been caused by the hiding of the pain. The pain is our honour and we are in awe of the pain and therefore we celebrate the pain and we do not hide the pain for it is time for the pain to be released and exposed for what it truly is.

> The pain of women that need not lie here anymore. We can release this pain and allow it be as the emblem of our true power, our true sense of women. We release this soul and allow her to continue in her work and to bring her light to the very many, many, women who are currently shrouded also under this fear of pain. We do not fear pain, we embrace the pain because it is our power. And through allowing this, the pain is no more. It is time for this soul to fly and to be free of this ancient pain that has held her back and held her down and we honour her with our love. And so it is.

So much of our physical pain and dis-ease is created through the emotional pain we carry, whether from this lifetime or others if the soul feels it necessary to. If we release ourselves from the individual pain, this has a powerful effect on the collective, for all women and our future children.

For me, Mary Magdalene's message also implies that the way our babies are birthed into the world also needs to be addressed. There is so much fear and so much money to be made around pregnancy, that pregnancy and birth has been medicalised to the point that the majority of midwives in America haven't been at a natural birth. At the time of writing in 2020, the state of maternity care took an even bigger nose dive to the point that midwives I know and trust were not calling it birth trauma, but obstetric violence. Women having to birth alone, fathers not allowed to be with and bond with their babies or support their wives in hospital after birth, pre-term babies separated from their mums and dads. Inductions for no other reason than it suited the hospital regime at the time. Horrifying for the women, my clients coming to terms with this gross disempowerment and a real question mark over our humanity. I had to keep reminding myself that these brave women and babies who experienced this were on a higher level, bringing up and out this consciousness of power over – particularly power over women. We continue to hold the light for change.

Because there are so many positive, incredible birth stories. So many women haven't experienced the pain of birth, only the joy in the pain – myself included at Samuel's birth. As Mary Magdalene says, our pain is our power, we are at our most powerful when conceiving, carrying, and delivering new life. Why then are so many asking us to hand over that power?

## For someone to have power over us, we have to allow it to be given

I am not anti-medical and am hugely grateful for it; myself and my boys may not be here without it. But there is surely a middle way where women are trusted with their sense of knowing, ancient knowing, heard and empowered during this most precious time and not surrounded by fear or that someone else knows best. If this balance shifts then both women's and babies' experiences shift to a much more positive outcome, which in turn changes the way they show up and view the world, which in turn, of course, changes the world. We're starting to fear the medical and that's not the best outcome either. Balance, always balance.

There's a lot to be said about the systems we're living in, whether that be fertility, maternity, education or governance. One way Rosa asked me to look at 'the system' was in gratitude. When I questioned this, she said, it is showing us exactly what wounds we are already carrying. Without it we may not be aware that we're not owning our power, or holding onto an energy of suffering, of being a victim etc. It is the system that is showing people not only their current situation, the frustrations, fear and power imbalance they hold about it – but the wounds that have been there for a very long time. Rosa showed me a time when they'll be no need for 'the system', because it won't be showing us anything. This was a complete reframe for me. Also bearing in mind that the people working in 'the system' are also bringing their ancient and current wounds to what they do. Imagine a world when more and more people are able to move into self-awareness and self-responsibility for how we feel and behave. This is where we're heading.

## 'A time of resolving trauma and restoring Truth'

Embracing and celebrating all of who we are as women, coming out of hiding and fear of judgement, is happening across the globe right now.

There are thousands of women throughout history and right now, recognised or unrecognised by the wider world and society, who have stood up and changed the world: Rosa Parkes, Marie Curie, Florence Nightingale, the suffragettes, Dorothy Vaughn (one of NASA's first women scientists), Reese Witherspoon, Mo Mowlam.

The list goes on and on and on. We all own the potential and power as individuals to rock the world; to transform the world. This is happening on a global scale energetically speaking. We are being offered the opportunity to rise to our full potential. Our journey to motherhood, whether challenging or not, is one access point.

The next few messages from Rosa offer a spiritual perspective of the bigger picture behind it all.

What is meant by the Divine Feminine and the Divine Masculine? Below is Rosa's insight into these two important energies. When brought into balance they enable the birth of a Divine Child – the Divine Child that is you.

### Rosa speaks of the Divine Feminine

What is the Divine Feminine? The Divine Feminine isn't simply about women. It is a principle that includes man and the birds and the bees for it is an energy, a presence, a consciousness in all and everything that you see around you and is in fact the consciousness of the very earth itself.

Do you see now the connection between the healing of the earth and the healing of yourselves? For as one heals so does the other. You humans always see life as one of material and matter and you do not take responsibility for what that matter actually is, which is, of course, energy, simply energy.

Many holes were made in the energy systems of your planet at some point in time and therefore this energy of love that had been held here for so long, not held in order to hold onto to, but held in order to have a place from which it could be shared, was in fact taken and hoarded and drilled and turned and replicated in other forms.

And this of course was seen eventually in the ways your earth was treated physically. The matter that is made up of your earth and all the crystals and the rocks and the seeds and the plants and the very magic in the soil itself was lifted and taken and used and abused and manufactured, and this is what we see is happening here on your planet today.

The energy of the earth itself, the Divine Feminine energy of love, of provision, of wealth and of abundance, of a love which knows no depths or feels no depths because it is infinite in its expression, has been laid waste by many centuries of abuse, of greed, by those who wish to harness it and mould it into their own expression, rather than the expression of what it truly is, which is the all and everything of the all and everything.

The Divine Feminine is an expression of love, an expression of unconditional love, which was bestowed upon the earth at the time of its creation that has slowly but surely been plagiarised, copied, taken and abused by the opposite of this expression, which is greed, anger and lack of. Do you see how this balance was tipped in favour of the opposite of the Divine Feminine energy – the masculine?

This is not to say that the masculine, the opposite, is bad, but do you see that the more the Divine Feminine expression was abused and distorted, so was the Divine Masculine expression of love and honour, support and regal loyalty?

The balance was tipped in the energies for the Divine Feminine to become softer and softer and more and more vulnerable and unable to withstand the increasing distortion of the male expression, which became ever more fuelled by anger and ego, lack and wanting, power over rather than power with for the greater good of all.

Do you see how all this happened, dear Debra? The poking of the holes into the Divine Feminine as she gave and gave and gave with everything she had out of a sense of wholeness, of strength of loving and of joy, only to have that quelled and questioned and taken by those who felt that it was unfair that one should have it and not all. Not realising that they did all indeed have it, but it was their own distorted ego which felt that they did not.

I am hoping this makes sense to you, my dearest Debra, for it is a level of understanding that perhaps goes back to the many times before now when deep inside the earth you were the one who was able to keep this flame of love alive in everyone and everything. And now it is so again and you will again see the light of Lemuria rising high above the shadows of the distortion that has taken place over the many lifetimes you have lived.

For the flame is once again lit and the fire of the earth will come alive once again to be seen by all and felt by all in order for the love to grow once again into the hearts of all men and all beings who choose to reside on this planet of yours, and indeed of all life beyond the reaches of the Mother that you call earth.

For this is indeed the heart of the universe and it is time for it to be known as such once again, through all the work and all the enlightenment that is taking place on this very special planet.

## Times are a-changing – the goddess message

Times are indeed a-changing and more balance is coming into the world. Women are rising up and allowing themselves to be fully seen in all of their wonder. The message below is from a collective of goddesses that I thought might be inspiring for you to read.

The Council of Light that is the female antithesis of the males is here to tell you that it is a time of change and that it is the rise of the female that is of the utmost concern and importance at this time. For just as there is a god there is an equal and actual counterpoint of balance within the goddess. And may all humans know that just as there is the male, there is an equal and actual counterbalance in the female.

It is now that this counterbalance is truly rising and rising to the forefront of consciousness as your women themselves begin to question and to reinterpret the musings of men from lifetimes ago.

For who indeed are the female protagonists of history? And who indeed is noticing that they are now beginning to come to the forefront of the minds? This is not a blame thing, or a cry, or a crime, but what is becoming ever more clear on your planet is that it will be a crime indeed in your terms, if this state of imbalance is allowed to continue.

We are asking our females of history, and of now, to recognise themselves as the new, as the one and the same. As the warrior princesses who went into battle, as the female creators and earth-bringers of the tribes, as the gods and goddesses of the modern day, to turn your land and to turn your earth once again into that place of Utopia, once again to the world of ubiquitous.

Into a world of flourishing beauty and presence, colour and grace, love and understanding from which all of humankind can flourish. And not simply the few, for which their control and their greed and their misunderstanding of how the world operates, has led to its demise.

No more our gods and goddesses, no more.

Your time is here, your time is now, your time has come. And rise you shall and rise you shall, bringing all others with you on your paths of enlightenment, on your paths of light.

The feminine is rising and bringing more balance. Inconsistencies in levels of pay between men and women, in business and in leadership positions, are being shown up ever more clearly. The image of the 1950s housewife at the beck and call of her husband is fading as both men and women awaken to the idea that women having the responsibility of 'keeping house' alone is utterly bonkers and unfair, and there is absolutely no reason for it, except for old ingrained patterns and beliefs carried down the generations that this is the way it should be.

There is a long way to go for old patterns of responsibility and what is 'women's work', and the sense of obligation that women feel to take on all the childcare and chores. But there has also been so much positive change with moves such as mums and dads now being able to share maternity leave so the dad has a chance to hang out with his children. And also questions of how a woman should or should not behave – or what it means to be a man. Women and children have been seen as commodities to be owned and there is still bride price in certain cultures. In the west, the tradition is that women are still 'given away' by their fathers to their husbands.

These are all constructs that have been imposed and lived in. They are changing because you are allowing yourself to see yourself more clearly. See your value as an individual more clearly, your desires and your own truth, finding your own box to fit in instead of trying to fit into somebody else's box and view of what life should be.

There is a wave of change within men and women as to how they see, and wish to live life, and a collapsing of those old beliefs. At some point in time, this wave will ride to every shore. The patterns we've seen over the last couple of generations clearly show the division between men and women, and in energy terms, the power play between the energies of the Divine Feminine and the Divine Masculine.

So, what lies beneath the need for men to feel the need to control and suppress women – to see women as less than? I asked Rosa about this.

### Rosa speaks of The Divine Masculine

The Divine Masculine is an energy of the highest order. It is one of the makers of creation, the makers of the universe, and along with the Divine Feminine, makes up much of the world's energy. It doesn't make up all of the universal energy though. As with everything, it is simply an aspect of all that is.

The Divine Masculine and Divine Feminine come together in love, the heart and soul, birth and death, power and softness, love and hate, black and white, the duality of existence of life here on your planet.

And it was this energy that took the action, that nurtured the creation of life on earth, that saw it spread and accumulate.

The Divine Masculine is the beautiful energy of the male, the planter and seeder of life, the bringer of life and harvester of life. It is an energy that is as harsh as it is loving: harsh in the sense of fiercely protective, not harsh in the sense of being hard, or being bad.

This harsh aspect, which is also carried in the feminine energy, became too much. The harsh energy of the Divine Masculine began to find excuses to be harsh, not out of love and not out of honouring the feminine, but out of honouring and protecting itself.

It began to find reasons in the form of the ego, of why they shouldn't have this or why they shouldn't have that. Instead of giving from love, the energy began to give from fear – fear that something was being taken from them, fear that they were being colluded into doing all that they did, not because this was the balance of the energies, but because this was the imbalance of the energies.

The parity of the all-powerful female whose ability to create and produce and the male to love and to serve as she did so was becoming out of balance. For who were these females who could just give and give and give and have no thought for the male who had to serve and serve and serve the goddess?

What was their role? What was their purpose? Were they not part of creation too? And yet they were not honoured for their part in creation; they were not recognised for the role that they were playing. The only way they were honoured was through the love of the female, the sex of the female.

The male decided it was time to take back some of their power, to take back some of their service to the Divine Feminine, to the goddess, and bring more balance, bring more love and bring more honouring to the male role in the serving of the goddess, the serving of the Mother, Mother Earth.

Yet, they could find no way to do so, so intent was the female on creating and so intent was the male on serving the female that the male could not keep up. The male could not find himself a space in the creation story, other than to serve.

This began to rile the male, and shake up the energy of the male as the ego began to question why them and not me. Why them to bring creation and why me to honour and serve. The ego began to question as to how it had come to this. How it had come to them doing all the work, doing all the honouring, and yet it was the goddesses who were praised and the goddesses who were honoured and the goddesses who were blessed with the ability to create.

They forgot that the male was the one who seeded the creation. The male forgot that it was he who was not offered love and sex as gratitude but offered love and sex because it was love and sex and the coming together of the male and the female that was necessary to seed life.

## Love and sex as the weapon of power

So it was that love and sex became a weapon of power. That if the women wished to create they could only do so at the will of the male and not at the love of the male. For the male had forgotten that they were not only here to serve but also to create.

They had forgotten that to create they were needed too. That love and sex were not handed to them out of pity, or with a pat on the head for being a 'good boy' and doing what they were told, they too were the creators of life. But they did not recognise this and they did not choose to remind themselves of this, for all they saw was the power and the magic of the female and all they felt were the scraps of love that were given to the male.

The males decided that the only way to bring themselves back into balance was to take what the female had, and that was love, sex, and creation. They began to recognise their own power in this game of life, it was they who began to diminish the sex of the female, they who began to wish to play a greater part in creation, by wounding the feminine, by ridiculing the sex they offered, by questioning their power of creativity. And, eventually, the balance of power shifted.

It is this fear of once again being the servant of the female that stops men from seeking out who they truly are at heart, and that is the creators themselves. The ones who carry the seed and the love that brings forth life in the female. But so anguished are they by the thought of their non-creation, by the thought of their non-ability to produce and to birth, they forgot their ability to seed and to nurture. They forgot their ability to create life, and once life has been formed, in their role as the teachers of life, of balance, alongside the female.

It is this remembrance, this honouring of their skills and abilities, this honouring of themselves of all of who they are and of all that they bring, to be reassured in their equal and balanced role in the continuing creation of life on earth, alongside their female counterpart.

It is so important to recognise this balance on all sides as the Divine Feminine continues to rise; that it is balance and not power or revenge, or being over the male, that is being recreated once again here.

For the female to step up into her role as the birther of life and the male to step up into his role as the protector of that life. A life that is not to be taken from for fear of being taken from, but a life that is to be given for the greatest good of all.

And so it is.

Take a moment to sit with the above messages and notice how they make you feel. How have you felt controlled or held back in your expression as a woman, and been affected, in particular, by the disempowerment that comes from experiencing such cruel challenges to your ability to become pregnant, to create? Or perhaps your own mother's ability to nurture, and the frustration, resentment and not feeling able to be her full self, plays out in your relationship with her.

Notice how this masculine fear of being inconsequential to creating life itself, which is buried so deeply and unconsciously, is playing out in terms of fear, lack and that something is being taken from them. Is this leading to the need to 'own' something and therefore to take and control? If I could draw a physical picture of what this fear looks like, within unimaginable depths of darkness, are scenes of all-out war. A sense of: you have more than me, so I'm going to take it.

Another way I see it playing out is when people feel that they own something or someone, but they are not so comfortable in owning it and they fear it may be taken from them, so they go to take more just in case. I also see it in people as a sense of having every right to take it, a justification of power over and survival of the fittest.

Remind yourself here that this is not a battle of the sexes. Do your best to stay out of blame. This is the ego, which is keeping you less than who you are. This is an inner conflict that lies within every woman and every man as we grapple with the hugeness of the wound of imbalance, the original wound that saw men in so much fear they began to need to control the mother, control the feminine, control creation and have power over. And the women so in fear of the shame and abuse, they found themselves giving away their power.

So, what will it feel like if we succeed as individuals and as a collective to heal our female sense of being less than and handing our power away because of it, and for men to heal their fear about being less than and taking power because of it? What will it feel like to achieve balance? And how do we do it?

**Rosa speaks about the Divine Child**

> The Divine Child, my dear, is you. The Divine Child is everyone reading this book. The Divine Child is every single human

on earth, even if you don't think they should or could hold the title of Divine. For the truth is, divinity isn't bestowed on you because you are good, just as hell isn't bestowed on you because you are deemed bad – it is a state of being. You simply are all Divine.

You can feel the power of that word, no matter what language you speak, because the word has an energy around it, just as you have spoken about the energy of names. So do you see yourself as a Divine Child? Do any of you see yourself as a Divine Child – the children of the Divine? Because that is what you all are, you and me both, we are all Divine for we are all made up of the same stuff, albeit put together in many different ways.

What is stopping you from seeing yourself as the Divine Child? What is it that makes you feel you are not worthy of Divinity? For it is not God who tells you this. It is not I who tells you this, and it is not even yourself who tells you this. It is the imbalance in energy and emotions that tells you this. For you have all been disconnected from your birth and from this truth for many eons of time, and it is time now to dispel the myths that you are not of the Divine and therefore not Divine, for this is simply just another tale in the long saga of the battle between the male and the female energies.

Most of you will have at one point in time been both the male and the female and therefore you carry the energy of this in your make-up, in your DNA and in your past, present, and future lives. It is simply who you are, a balance of the two, alongside the many other energies that make up this great experience of being human. This great play of being in a human body and living in a human life.

For you all of course hold the energies of the angelic realms, the galactic realms, the peaceful realms, and the earth realms within you. It is simply a matter of unlocking them. I do not take this lightly when I say 'simply' because I know it is not simple and does not feel simple from your human point of view, because you have all been witness to and experienced much of what is wrong in your world.

Some of you have turned off these strands of yourself out of fear and as a protection to keep you safe from the harm of those who couldn't bear to be near such a presence of light and freedom from control.

For others, these strands have been turned off for you. Imagine these strands as cords of light that keep you connected to your energy body, all of your energy bodies, that keep you connected to Source. It is in this connection to Source through these strands that you will find your self, find your Divinity, for then you will know yourself to be connected, simply connected.

Again, I do not use this word 'simply', lightly, for what can be so simple about connection, particularly to the Divine when you so often find it hard enough to connect with yourself as you connect with others in your human world? How are you to find this connection to the other world, the other strands of life that surround you whether seen or unseen?

For the seen I mean the earth, nature and the nature spirits of animals and creatures, as well as the strands of connection to others. For the unseen I mean the strands to the realms of the angels, the Masters, the commanders, and the realms of the starseeds, the seeders of the planets that helped to seed the earth and therefore helped in seeding you in your human self.

So, to start your imaginations, imagine all of those golden strands of light moving through your body, moving in your cells, and any that are not flowing, pick off the lid that is holding them shut, for this is a lid that is no longer necessary. It is a lid that is keeping you from your connection, keeping you from your belief and knowing in your own divine self.

There are many reasons these are in place. It is of no consequence what they may be, unless you choose to go deeper and to find out. For now, just see the lids and imagine allowing yourself to know what it feels like to take them off. Allow your full connection to the truth of you to flow through.

How does it feel? All of us here in the higher realms were able to lift off these seals over very many lifetimes of learning to live with them. We now are living without them. It is that some of us choose to stay in those higher realms and some of us choose to re-enter earth without the seals, or at least without as many of them.

You now are already the Divine Child, albeit with your lids on, which are slowly and gently being lifted off as is your will and is your right. Yet the spirit babies who are coming to you are deciding to come back to you, back to earth, with fewer of these lids and seals in place, for they wish to know and remember much quicker their divinity and their connection to all things.

They too are the Divine Children coming in to help seed the New Earth, be the New Earth, with their connection already in place and remembered, or for some reminded of them, of this, by you, their parents of light.

The Divine Child is really one of feeling fully connected, fully open to the life-force energy of the earth and the sun, the moon and the stars and the heavens themselves. It is all there for you if you choose to look. It is all here for you if you choose to look. It is all here for you, happening for you, right now, in this moment if you choose it to be so.

So, what is it that you are choosing? Are you choosing the disconnection in order to feel safe from harm or judgement? Or are you choosing connection to keep you safe from harm or judgement? Whichever way you choose is the choice for you. It is for you to know that you are the children of light, the children of the Divine, the Divine Child at all times, whether you believe it to be true in this moment or not.

Within all of this, you are loved unconditionally, for all that you are and all that you bring to this beautiful planet called earth.

And so it is.

I admit it takes me a while to absorb and understand the messages. Feel into your own reading and meaning of them – there are many layers to them depending on where you are on your 'awakening' journey. If I was to summarise them at the level of understanding I have now, it is that we are all of course Divine, from the same Divine source, and each with a magnificent role to play – whether that is deemed to be a good or bad role, it is a necessary and Divine role. I also get the impression we are all living and re-living time and time again, lifetime after lifetime, the ancient wound of the mother – the wound of the feminine having her power taken and the fear of the masculine driving the need to be powerful – as the male and female energies became so out of balance eons ago.

It doesn't feel fair that we are having to experience so much suffering and so many challenges in our fertility journey, in our life journey in the here and now, because of something that happened however many years ago. But this is when we have to remember we likely played a part in it. We are all effectively recycled, coming back time and time again to remember who we truly are, which is Divine, which is love. And if we don't do our own inner work to heal the aspects of this wound that we individually carry, then we will continue to be living in it on a personal level and collectively.

The more of us who wake up, the more the scales tip back into balance. The souls waiting to come in, in hordes, have likely lived this many times and are in a position to come back, as Rosa says, with the lids off, with the veils off, with this knowing of their Divinity, and therefore they will be less likely to get pulled into society's judgements and ways of doing things. They will bring change because they simply won't think or feel as we did as children, or do now. Their self-knowing won't be as deeply buried as perhaps ours was, or is.

This is why they are encouraging us to do our inner work, to help them remember, to recognise their Divinity and their role in building a New Earth, a new way of seeing and operating in the world that isn't one of control and lack but of oneness, cooperation, and balance.

How special are you to be the ones they have chosen to help and guide them with this? At a time when you are potentially feeling at your worst, a failure, undeserving, a victim of life, please, please know that on some level you are ancient enough, wise enough, strong enough, courageous enough and loving enough to be able to face the heart of your wounds, the ones you are living with every day, and the much deeper underlying ones held in your soul and your DNA.

As I was editing this chapter a friend happened to send me a poem by Karen Star on the feminine. She writes of how the feminine will not surrender to the wounded masculine who belittles, controls, manipulates, dishonours, abuses or attacks her. And only surrender to the Divine Masculine who elevates, Honours, Cherishes, Supports and protects her. It's within this space she will feel safe enough to fully give of her mind, body, heart and soul. This is the dance of love and balance of the polarities within and with another.

An interesting message about the spiritual perspective of IVF is one way of demonstrating how this imbalance in the energy within and without is being shown to us. The deeper I have gone into the messages, the more I've realised that literally everything is showing us the bigger picture, giving us clues to what is going on, shouting at us to heal the imbalance. I can't find the words, but 'illusion' springs to mind. Almost like we're puppets being played if you choose to look at it that way, or alternatively and more helpfully and empowering, directors of the play where we get to choose the next scene.

**Rosa on the spiritual perspective and bigger picture of IVF**

IVF is simply a process, yet another process, in which your baby souls are enabled to connect in with you in physical form. There has been much damage to the female psyche in the form of power and control that men and science have put upon them in their unconscious bid to control the creative process. In this psyche are beliefs such as: I need help to conceive, I need help to create, I cannot create alone and also I am in no position to create without the power of the male, the power of the man, the power of the masculine.

Do you see how the psyche of women has been damaged over such a long period of time? To the point where they believe, mostly unconsciously, they cannot create, should not create, unless there is some form of control coming in from the masculine energy?

That it is in the handing over of power to another that will enable them to create. This is a huge hole in the psyche of women, the psyche of the female and the psyche of the feminine, because they believe on some very deep and unconscious level that they are not allowed to create unless they are given the chance to by another.

Do you see how this is playing out in your world of loss of control, of power in and power over the female? For it is not only useful for the man, the masculine, to have this control over creation, but also for the women, for the feminine, to be in a position of being subservient to it. This is often deemed as safer, more respectable. It is often deemed as the way it should be with the power of the women to create taken and given this blessing through the power of the man, the masculine, to enable this to happen.

This is not to blame the woman for being in this psyche, nor is it to blame the man, yet it is time now to look at these deep-seated patterns of betrayal that your process of IVF brings up in both women and men. For it is often the male of the species who cannot procreate and therefore is in need of assistance to help bring this to fruition. This too is a reflection of the damage to the psyche when their own feminine nature has been dampened to such an extent that they no longer feel able to even take up the male's role in creation, the seeding.

Do you see that IVF is your human ingenious way of helping to create life whilst avoiding the very reason why life is not being created in the first place – which is through the meeting of the power of the woman and the love of the man for her. This union of the male and the female.

IVF was created by and within the masculine energy to circumnavigate this wound, this fear of being inconsequential to the creation process, by offering an alternative to going in and witnessing the damage created in the female psyche through years, generations, of abuse for being able to create. That women must create this way in order to appease the male, in order to keep him assured that the woman isn't all-powerful in the first place. That she too needs help to create and that help comes in the form of the masculine energy that surrounds your science.

This science of yours is a great thing, a noble thing and a much wished-for thing, for all of it comes from the inspiration of men and women of good heart, good faith and good inspiration to circumnavigate the 'problems' of nature.

Yet, we are also asking for some balance within this science and this balance will come when the deep-seated fears of the feminine that we are too powerful, too special, too much, and that we are not allowed to be, for this makes the life of another uncomfortable when they believe that they are not all-powerful, loving and creative.

We do not wish to upset the other because often this other has brought us harm. Harm in the physical sense and harm in the greater sense of reducing us to nothing more than an object to be used or adorned.

This is the power and the imbalances of the male and female energies. And your IVF is one way that this is being played out.

## Babies come in spite of IVF not because of it

Babies come because they wish to come and they wish to be with their parents and this is a beautiful and loving thing, a moment of pure joy and creation. No woman should feel less than if she has welcomed her baby through IVF, because her baby has arrived because they love each other. Her baby has arrived because she has loved herself enough to be put through this most highly disturbing science. Her baby soul is her baby soul no matter which way they arrive and no matter their journey to coming into the world.

However, it is in spite of and not because of the science of IVF. In these words, women should take heart of their own power and their ability to create because it was not the IVF that brought their baby to them but they who brought their baby to them.

This may not make sense to those who have welcomed their baby through IVF for, of course, they are grateful for the science that allowed this physical act to come to fruition. But please read my words carefully, feel them deeply. It is in spite of the IVF process and not because of it that your baby soul came to you.

You must know that it is your power to create that birthed them into life and not the power of the medical, the power of the man. The masculine energy that seems to dominate your world in all aspects of life, including the medical and scientific. So please take heart all of you women who are going down this route of IVF, for those of you who have yet to meet them in physical form – it is you – it is always you who hold the power to create, to hold the life-force energy of another and to grow and nurture that life form into the home of your baby soul.

It is not the physical, it is you. If you are entering into this process in order to meet your baby, do so with an open mind as to your own power, your own right to create, for that is what you are here for – to create life: your life, as well as the life of another if that is part of your soul's wishes.

Do not hand over your power to the science and the medical. Be in the power of you as you utilise the inspiration and the genius of the science and the medical but always be in no doubt that it is you who are the creator.

We implore you to know this for the damage to the female psyche in the act of creation is so ingrained, so deep, that it must be addressed sooner rather than later. If your baby is coming to you now then it is always worth remembering to go back to your IVF journey at some point and be curious about how you felt, question how you saw yourself within it. Question the very heart of you in this process, as you are not handing yourself over to the God of science in order to bring your baby into your arms. You are still, and always will be, handing yourself over to the God-ness of you, the goodness of you, the heart of you and your right and heartfelt wish and desire to create.

For this can so easily be taken from you during your IVF process as the most miniscule of physical changes are logged and opinionated about. If this the case, admire your body for all of its changes and its numbers and its high this and low that, for isn't that the miracle of the body in and of itself, that it is able to experience the ups and downs of all its life aspects – much as you do.

Be fascinated by the figures, be amazed by the numbers, but do not judge the numbers. Do not make the numbers and the opinions of others make you feel small, make you feel ashamed of your body. Be in awe of your body for it will carry the life force of your baby soul. If you allow it to do so, know it can do so.

If your body can change as dramatically and as often as the results so too can it change dramatically to the physical results that you wish to see; the numbers that your doctors feel comfortable with seeing. It is your mind where you can ease the harm from these results instead of fearing them. You can do this by going into the psyche, the energy, the form and the body of you to change the way you wish to feel about creation, and yourself as the creator.

Do you hear me, our women of light? Do you hear what I am saying? That you are the light. You are the power and you are the healer of your own self and the selves of many, way back down in your own timelines. You are the saviours of women because you have the power to create even when you have been told you cannot. You are the saviours of women because the more you heal and transform your own conscious and ancient, hidden memories of being harmed for being a creator, you too are healing the psyche of women everywhere.

At no time in history has there been more need, more desire, for processes such as IVF, and I ask you: why is this? Is this because women are beginning to stand in their power and demand the right to create life? Or is it that this harmful energy of not being allowed to create, not being able to create, not being good enough, strong enough or worthy enough to create, is now coming up to be seen? Seen so it can be called out for what it is: a pain, a trauma, a damage, a hurt, that is a long time in coming to be recognised as such. To be recognised as the very original wound of the mother, that of your ability, power and specialness to create new life.

A knowing and a right that has been subjugated, dismissed, and derided as 'women's work' and all because of the underlying fear about just how powerful we truly are.

For all you women going through IVF, I am with you, with heartfelt love. Whether before you begin the process, or when you are in the process, or a long time after the process, I ask you to step into the truth of what is happening, the truth of you, the truth of miracles, the truth of love, the truth of the creative power you are, despite what you may feel or have been told.

I ask you now to clear away all things that are not aligned with this truth. For this is the next stage of evolution and you are very much a part of it.

And so it is.

Fertility struggles, baby loss, and birth trauma can all be incredibly disempowering. The way I read Rosa's messages is that for those of us on a very challenging, disempowering, and seemingly 'out of your control' journey to motherhood, your task is to reclaim, or at least begin to reclaim, your sense of self. Know, feel and believe the power that lies within you as a woman. Delve in and see those parts of you that hold onto the wounds from this lifetime, and others, so you can transform them and reclaim the power of the feminine, the Divine Mother, in order to restore yourself, others, and the earth back into balance.

This theme of empowerment and reclaiming a sense of self runs through all of my client sessions. It always made sense. It makes sense to us all to want to feel the best we can feel and not at the mercy of anyone else or life itself, but instead know what our boundaries are and know we have a choice how to move through life. Learning to say no to things that don't bring you joy and yes to you and your joy.

Through writing this book I now know, and I hope you do too, just how key this is to your future, your children, future children, and the future of all. It is not about power over someone or something. It is not about allowing anyone else to make choices for you or put you under pressure to make choices that make you give your power away. True power is actually peace. True power is peaceful because there is no inner conflict. True power is knowing and believing in your 'self' without holding onto the wounds of the past that you know or don't know about.

I read a quote from Jonathon Larson that says: "the opposite of war is not peace, it's creation." The way I read this is, when we are not at war with ourselves, when we are balanced, we are in an optimal place to create – able to flow more easily in the creative energies.

So what is this energy of power from a higher perspective? I asked Rosa.

### Rosa on the theme of power

Power. Today I would like to share about the concept of power. What does power mean to you? Because from where

I'm sitting, I have been watching you give your power away to others for many eons, because you have been scared by their power. But how can you be scared of a power that has been taken – because is that not essentially yours? Is it your power you are scared of?

We ask you at this time to take your power back; to ask yourself who is in charge of you? Who is in charge of your life? Who is in charge of your time? Your finances? Your freedom? Your world?

How is it that others hold you in their power, through their taxes and their police, through their religious claims and their cultural norms? Are these norms for you? Are they your ideals and dreams and wishes or do they simply happen because it is easier to allow someone else your power? Is it easier to act like an automaton and to ridicule and humiliate those who are not of this same like mind in order to ease the pressure on yourself and the guilt of knowing that you, neither, are in charge of you?

How can we help you to find your power? What is it that you can do to recognise, feel, to be brave and courageous and to say no to the systems that have kept you from experiencing the delights of your manifestations instead of the traumas and the cyclical rounds of the ups and downs of life from which the effects are largely of others' making?

This is because you are basing your reality on that of others and not of your 'selves'. We ask you now to look at which aspects of life you feel are not in your power. Which aspects of life you are running for the pleasure and convenience of another and not of your 'self'.

In so doing, you will become aware of the changes that you can make in order to empower yourselves. Do you see that because I am you and you are me, I am them and they are you, and that by allowing yourself the pleasure of being who you are and reclaiming that aspect of yourself, you are allowing others to do the same?

And so the collective becomes one of not working for the love of another or for the whim of another but for the power of the 'self', and the self is always and forever the self of self-love and the self of the Divine.

## The self

Reading the messages above, you will draw your own conclusions. For me, I think I've got the message and insight that we are the Divine Feminine, we are the Divine Masculine, we are the Divine Child. (As an aside we are also much more than this, a lovely mix of many energies from many realms but we're focusing on these two energies for now). By recognising these aspects of ourselves and what each offer, and bringing all of the parts of you – the hurt parts and the loving parts, the battling, inner-conflict parts – back to oneness, to wholeness, brings you to the 'self'.

Through your 'self' is your power; your 'self' is the hugeness and love that you are. Re-discovering your 'self', mastery of your 'self', through joy I may add, is just the little task you've set yourself! It's not a one lifetime mission and likely it's taken lifetimes to get to where you are now in terms of self-awareness and self-love and self-belief. It's more important than ever to declare yourself as a sovereign being.

## Being selfish or assertive

One question I used to grapple with is: if it's all about the self, then firstly, isn't that selfish? I've realised this is even more conditioning, a limiting belief, one that holds on very tightly. It serves some people to accuse you of being selfish by thinking and doing what's right for you, because you're not pandering to their needs and wants.

It's not being selfish; it's being assertive and is a necessity. Not only for your well-being and growth but for others' too. Because if you're not filling them up and giving them whatever they think they need and want, then they'll have to start taking responsibility for themselves and their own choices and finding out what it is they truly need.

Women, in particular, are trained to be unselfish and through the messages so far you can see where the root of it comes from – another form of control which taps into our unconscious sense of being unworthy. Saying no and being assertive are certainly something to practise because the belief that we shouldn't be selfish runs very deep, and they don't come easily! But you absolutely can begin to play with this. Try being assertive on for size and notice how it makes you feel. It doesn't mean not caring. It doesn't mean not helping or being kind. It means if it doesn't feel right and you're doing something out of obligation or because you 'should', then perhaps it's time to bring out that loving no.

If it helps, when you do something for someone out of obligation, think about the energy you're actually giving them. You may be giving them something practically, but the energy behind it is not coming from love. Wouldn't the most loving thing be to say yes to yourself first; fill up your own cup and the overflow of you and what you give has a very different energy around it. The person you're giving to will feel that love.

As a woman going through a testing journey to motherhood, remember from the IVF message the absolute hugeness of what you are healing and transforming, because you have the love, power, and strength to do so, even if that's not how you feel. Knowing this, don't you think you have every right to mind yourself? Every right to conserve every ounce of strength for yourself? This is big work you are doing. Do what's right for you.

Which brings me to another question I have grappled with. How is that by being selfish, or I prefer 'assertive', we can help the collective? Each of us is, of course, an individual, a unique soul with our own unique life experiences and vibration – but we are also part of the collective, because we are all connected. We are all from the same source, as you will read in Part 3 of this book. But only you can heal yourself. Only you can make the choices you need to create change in your life. Only you can hold the energy of you and the energy of your baby. There will be many people who cross your path who can guide you, but ultimately, it's you who has to make the choice and do the work. It's you who creates your life and what you are experiencing, whether you judge it to be a good or bad creation.

When you create out of love and not out of fear, when you find the courage to move through your wounds and free yourself by coming to a different perspective, you feel empowered and resilient. And when you feel revived, the people around you do too.

Have you noticed if you go into work and someone is not quite themselves and having a grumpy day how that affects you and the team? Even if they are not outwardly grumpy, you just sense there's something up. Like yawning, energy spreads – and the clearer and more congruent you become in your own energy, the more cohesion you feel within, the quicker you heal personally and the more positive vibes you spread. If you're happier, those closer to you are more likely to feel happier and then the people they hang out with that day get a chance to pick up some happy vibes too, and so on.

I love the phrase, from spiritual teacher Ram Dass, "We're all just walking each other home", home being the knowing of our true selves, the knowing that we are all pure love, coming from the source of pure love. We are each a unique jigsaw piece in a vast connected puzzle.

Knowing yourself is what is being asked of us by the future souls coming to earth so we can best guide them to remember that they are love. But in this bigger picture, and outside of conception, knowing ourselves and creating our lives is pretty much what we're here to do. That is our ultimate goal.

**Below is a message from Source about the nature of the self**

> Who of you here is aware of the self? Do you know who or what the self is? How it feels, what it needs, what it desires, how it wishes to be?

This is not the ego-self of psychology, but of the self that is the I am. The I am of the I am. The I am that is great, the I am that is lordly, the I am that is a picture of Divine Feminine or Masculine, or neither, or both, for the self is far from concerned about the gender of a person, or the identity of a person.

It has no concern for what you do or don't do, what you have or don't have, what is your life or what is your death. It has no concern for much at all, and even the word concern is not of concern to the self.

For the self has no concern. The self is all and everything of the all and everything of who you are. It makes no matter if you are a man or a woman; no matter if you are a child or an animal; and no matter if you are dead or alive. It is simply you – the eternal you that lives on, grows, learns, changes – which is always an illuminating presence in the world.

Do you see, as you strive and grow towards being the best version of yourself, it makes no matter, for you are already and are always that very best version of yourself.

You are always merely your self. What is it that drives you back to that self, drives you back into that place of remembering that you are and always have been perfect? You may well be on very different and unique paths in life, and yet for all of you, the aim is the same.

The aim is to remember, the aim is to learn and grow through your particular life experiences in order to get closer and closer to return to your God self – the ever-perfect and everlasting part of you that is the all and everything of the all and everything.

Is it time to forgive yourselves for all those times when you felt less than perfect? Is it time to know and understand that you already are what you wish to become? And in doing so, may this realisation, from the words of God himself and with the love of God herself, bring you into a sense of peace, a sense of relaxation, a sense of knowing that all and everything you have ever done, ever witnessed and experienced, is forgiven, is healed, is started anew, is ended and completed at each and every moment you make it a choice for it to be so.

For this is your power and this is your perfection and this is the beauty and the godliness of your self.

Not of me, for all I am is simply you, in all my guises and all my creeds and colours, my sex and desires, my needs and wants, my 'goodness' and 'badness', and you could not get this much perfection if you too were not already perfect.

For are you all not simply a reflection of the M E? The M E that is the miracle everlasting. The M E that is my everything. The M E that is the magic enduring – the magic and majesty of all of life in all its forms of which you are that.

As you see this perfection and the perfection in all things, then you will truly see yourself. And this is all I ask, for you to see your self.

It is time to love yourselves, for as and when you do this, you are loving all of ME. And for all of your trying and all of your striving and your human struggles, can you see that it is never your self that is struggling, but merely your desire to get back to your self in ways controlled by the mind of the ego-self and not of your ME self?

And so it is.

Just a little reminder here that there's no competition here as to how far along in your journey you are to self or to being in your power. I, for one, am not 'living' these messages right now. I may know the theory and the concepts, I may understand them to a certain level, but putting them into practise as a human being is a whole other ball game. We have to forgive ourselves for being human, we're doing the best we can with what we know. And then we learn and we grow.

I know I feel more my 'self' than ever before, like myself, even love myself, which was a place I never imagined I'd get to and I can't wait to feel more of this. I know I no longer people please as much as I used to but I also know I have a long way to go to fully 'be' empowered and self-loving. But that's the fun of life, the playground of earth we're in, and if we can make it as playful as possible, how different it would all feel. There are serious moments and situations and exploring your innermost thoughts and feelings can feel challenging and serious, but soul growth, becoming self-aware is not necessarily a serious business. The light beings I channel are playful, funny; these energies are light and bring light. The more we can laugh at ourselves, the easier and more likeable we find ourselves, the easier life is.

Admittedly, sometimes on this soul journey, there are times that are easier than others, when everything feels in flow and you're like: great, I'm in it! And then something else pops up that doesn't feel comfortable and off you go again, back to the healing drawing-room. The more you know and the more self-aware you are, the more you want to know. That's so exciting and when you feel different about something you haven't felt comfortable with or understood, you feel amazing, more free than you ever imagined. But as you rise, you also feel and experience more and become more aware of what doesn't feel right for you, and that includes the people you hang around with.

There are times I've thrown my hands up and shouted out to the Universe: what more do I need to know, what else can you possibly want me to do? Why can't I just be allowed to stay in the happy, loved-up feeling, why does something else always have to spring up such that I need to look at myself again? Sometimes, I want to forget about all this soul stuff and just go back to being Debra who worked for a charity, came home, played with the boys, cooked dinner, had a glass of wine, chatted to my husband and friends about nothing much in particular and went to sleep, rinse and repeat the next day. Sometimes that feels like such a relief. And so that's exactly what I do, because why not?

You're not in a race, all is perfect. When you need a rest from trying to figure it all out, rest, be and do whatever feels like the least amount of pressure, remember you're here to experience joy, you are joy. You have all the time in the world to experience you. This doesn't mean you've given up or gone backwards, that's impossible, you're just resting. Have no doubt your soul will be calling you before too long to start being curious again about your why and you'll feel ready to take that next step or leap. This message below from Source looks at why we have these soul callings to get to know ourselves more.

## Why is it so important to know your self?

If you know the self, your self, then you know ME. For this is all of who I am and as more and more of you come back to this understanding then the more and more we grow and come together – all as pieces of the same very large puzzle. As we start to recognise each other as such, as a different part of the same puzzle , then will we not begin to see that it is much more comfortable to have a piece of you beside you, rather than a piece of you who is against you?

A piece of you who feels that they do not fit, that they are not worthy and therefore not part of our puzzle and therefore they choose to destroy this puzzle in order that they don't feel left out of it.

Do you see how this may happen? This feeling left out, this feeling of not belonging, this feeling of the need to attack the self? Is it not their misunderstanding of the self that creates this divide? The misunderstanding of who they are and where they are; their need to belong and their need to fit in that is out of balance with the love that comes from knowing the self and knowing that all selves are indeed one and the same?

The more we are helped to understand the self, and the more we help others find their way back to self, then the picture of Utopia from which we have all come and which we all wish to create, can indeed be created in your lifetime, in your planet and beyond.

And so it is.

In the above message from Source, this energy speaks of ME. Who or what is this Me? The story of creation that I was shown appears in the third and final part of this book. Before we go there, it would be helpful if we start with the question: is there a God?

The very word brings up all sorts of emotions and triggers and means different things to different people, all of which are unique, depending on your life experiences, your culture and your upbringing. It is not the word, it is the energy around this word that is unique to each of you. I still rarely say the word God. It brings up too much conditioning around religion and I wasn't even brought up in a religious household. To my conditioned mind I go immediately to the Bible and patriarchal stories that God is a man, God is all-powerful, God punishes and you have to be good to know God. You can see who these stories serve and it certainly isn't ME, the individual.

This story of God comes from a place of fear, not love. So who am I 'talking' to when I ask to connect in with Source energy? What is the energy of clarity, or peace or fulfilment, of nothingness that I connect into when I'm meditating? No matter what healing work or channelling I'm doing, I always go to Source energy first – I see it as pearly iridescent light, brighter than the sun, or sometimes like the hugest, golden or red sun. It doesn't matter how you see it, it is the energy of unconditional love. There are no stories in this energy, no sense of deserving or un-deserving. It simply is love.

So here is a message from the source of unconditional love from which we all came.

# Is there a God?

## Message from Source/God/Creator

Let's talk about ME today, shall we? Who am I? What is my purpose? What is it that I bring you, each and every one of you?

Is it the death and destruction you are all so keen on talking about? Or is it the famines and the plagues and the demise of the human? Oh, the joys of being God and having this world, my world, my universe as my playground to come and do as I please, when I please.

As this is what many of you think of Me. That I am the cause of all your ills. How can I possibly allow all of this death and destruction on your planet? As well as being the cause of your joys.

I am here to tell you that it is time to wake up. Wake up, my sweet children of light, because this is what you are. And as each and every one of you experiences Me in your lives, it is only a short step for you to take to realise that I am nothing more and nothing less than you, your selves.

Am I blaming you now for all the ills in the world? No, no, this is not the case. For just like me, the world is your playground too and you are free to play and create and add your toys and games, add your essence out into the world as I do – for am I not simply a reflection of you?

If I am only a mere reflection of you, then what is it that you will do to change your worlds, to change your fates, to change your wishes and create and command at will – just as you believe I do?

For I am not outside of you. I am not separate from you, and so I cannot and will not allow you to see yourselves as such. And it often pains me to see you blaming me for the ills of the world, not because I am hurt, but because you are.

You do not see your selves as I see you, and therefore you do not see Me. How can it have reached such a point that you cannot see love? See the love that is you, around you, made of you? The love in the earth and the skies, the love in the food you eat, the plants you grow, the animals you kill and the earth you destroy?

Can you imagine, even for a short moment in time, that you see your selves as I see you? That you see me as I am, which is indeed you. That you can imagine, that you see and feel and hear and touch the love that is all and everything of your planet, that is all and everything of you?

The time for blame is now over. The time for passing the buck, whether that be to a politician, or a boss, a husband or a wife, a friend or a foe, this is no more. This is your world, this is your life, and it is time to see that you are indeed the God of it.

Your unique essence is in this world of love, made with love, and I ask you this now: in which way would you wish to see your world? If it is death and destruction – so it is that death and destruction you will make.

For you can no longer be seen as children of the church, or children of the services, or children of anything other than children of the light. Children of love. You are the light and it is you who have a choice to bring that light out into the world.

It is not for Me or for anyone else to tell you what it is to think, or to do, or to be, for it is imperative now that you know it is you who are the creator of your destiny and you who are the creator of your dreams.

All I ask is for you to see this, know this, take responsibility for this and make your choice in full knowledge that the dreams are yours and belong to no one or no thing else – but yours and yours alone.

It is time for you to know your power and to learn how to use this power wisely in order to create the world you wish to live in. And I implore you to choose well, my children, but it is not in my power to do anything other than give you your power to do exactly as you choose and therefore create that world that you choose.

In light. Your servant that is God.

Where Part 1 of this book explored the theme of creation from an individual perspective, of you as the woman, the man, and the baby, Part 2 has opened us up more to the idea of not so much physical men and women but the energies that we all carry no matter our gender; the energies of the feminine and the masculine. The messages offer us a perspective as to why we may be experiencing our lives the way we are, what is driving our choices, situations, and what we see happening in the world. Ultimately it reveals how an imbalance between these two energies is affecting our ability to create, to be in our full creative power as physical men and women.

Again, this may be enough information for you to mull over for now and be curious how you feel about what you've read so far. Does it feel true? Far from the truth? Perhaps something to be curious about and open to seeing how these energies are playing out in your own life? Wherever you're at is perfect. We are all being asked to find our own truth in how we see life because we've had centuries of being told what we should or should not believe; very often punished for not going along with the beliefs that society, culture and religion were aiming to put on us. It's time for the Self. When you know yourself, you come to a place of self-belief. With self-belief you don't fear judgement and you can better understand and support others. With self-belief, anything is possible. No one is limiting you. Imagine this world of freedom of self?

## Further expanding your awareness of the universe

As we move into Part 3 of the book, it's time now to expand your awareness again to the even bigger picture. The bigger picture of who you are, how you came to be, how the universe, the planets and earth came to be – creation itself – and the magnificent role you and each of us play to support the collective and the universe. Yes, it really is that big and, yes, you really are this powerful!

Much like growing up, we need to work up from figuring stuff out from our individual perspective to then realising the consequences of our actions on others. Only then do we see the bigger picture.

Part 3 of this book is the section I've been most hesitant about. I feel the messages, I get them, I 'see' them. What I see is our interconnectedness and how the universe works but the messages also blow my mind a little as the picture really is huge.

The purpose of me sharing is to join in the debate with others who have opened up or are opening up to the bigger picture and offer another perspective. They don't need to be your truth or the truth – just the information I've received to add into the mix of life with the intention of lifting humanity into their sense of magic, wonder, and magnificence. I'm a woman who, for whatever soul reason, is a messenger here to share these messages whilst – in my own human way – figuring them out, figuring life out, and living it the best way I can. Every one of us is a beautiful piece of a ginormous puzzle and each of help another to unlock more of the piece they are. Working together, the puzzle begins to come together.

These messages are here for everyone, no matter where you're at in your spiritual journey. If you're relatively new to these concepts, allow the messages to open up your mind to possibility. To bring a sense of the hugeness, vastness and magnificence of you, which is so much greater than what you've ever been told. I'm often told by spirit that I/we take life too seriously. There are serious challenges and issues that we face but life is not intended to be serious. Our aim is joy. Life is a game we're all trying to figure out and the more playful we can be with it the more joyful it feels, and the more we're in the energy of creation.

So, if stories of the universe, portals, planetary communication, earth spirits and galactics are not in your vocabulary as yet, read on as if reading from a sci-fi book or watching a Marvel movie and soak up the possibility and healing magic of the words without needing to figure them out. Or perhaps it's time for you to complete the book for now and head straight to the conclusion. Wherever you're at, it's with love that we now dive ever deeper into the universe and our place and connection to it and with it.

In Part 3 you'll read the 'story of creation' as told to me by Rosa, you'll get to know the earth on a much more intimate level with messages from those I call the earth spirits, with the intention of bonding with her, and therefore yourself, on a much deeper level, moving from separation to unity. We look at what drives war and conflict, what is joy, what are the underlying reasons for how the world has been and is, and why it's changing and moving into the New Earth energies, as are you. There are more insights on what this huge picture has to do with fertility and your journey to motherhood and the deep, spiritual significance of adoption.

Part 3 also flips certain stories we've been told upside down, offering another perspective, for example, why certain words that started off with such deep, beautiful meaning of the feminine have been corrupted into something derogatory. Why birthing has been 'taken over' by the masculine, medical model from the realm and sacred space of the feminine. Always ask who told you something, and why. Find your own truth.

However relevant worldly events feel to you, this next part of the book gives insight into why we see and experience the world as we do and reveals how big a part you play in bringing about balance. You are not separate from the world, from the earth, from others; you are All. You are love.

Delve into Part 3 with an open mind for some treats of insight and healing.

I feel Part 3 will at some point expand into a book in its own right, as I expand into the messages myself. There are so many more to share that don't feel quite right to add into this particular book, I'm not ready and maybe the world's not ready for them yet.

But here we are now, and here you are: Part 3 is the story of creation from Rosa's perspective and how we are all a part of it.

# Part THREE

# Chapter 12
## Rosa's Story of Creation
### Signs from the universe, war and peace, adoption and healing the wound of separation

It may seem odd to begin the end of this book with the story of the beginning of life, a creation story about the birth of the universe, but keep in mind Rosa's opening line in this book: There is no beginning or no end to this story, merely where I choose to start. We are all energy, never-ceasing energy that continually changes form. Essentially, this book is about the energy of creation.

What you have experienced, or are experiencing, on your journeys to motherhood, is how you as an individual are experiencing the energy of creation, of creativity and the imbalance and distortion of this energy. As Rosa says in one of her messages below, we need to know the root of why something is happening. It's then we can begin to change.

The information I'm about to share only came through once I'd started to write this book. As I mentioned, the idea for this book was given to me by Rosa in 2016. I thought then that it would be a powerful book to help women heal from the pain that challenging journeys to motherhood can inflict. Even this seemed like the bigger picture. But oh no, there is more, much, much more to it than that.

Just as it had taken me two years to get to the stage of feeling ready, feeling able, feeling safe enough I guess, to share my story and Rosa's messages and feeling very at peace with that, guess what? In she comes with even more mind-blowing information that threw me straight back into that fear of judgement and of being visible; the fear of sharing these big spiritual messages out into the world.

For whatever reason, I as a soul signed up to come and do exactly this, together with Rosa. According to my soul alchemist friend Marina Beech, who works in the Akashic Records, my spiritual gift is communication. I truly hope I am honouring this gift.

As I started to write this book, I read and re-read Rosa's messages. The more inner work and clearing I did, and conditioning I let go of, the more I began to understand the depth of her words.

Statements such as: "We are going to heal the world with this book, you and I, as we are going to bring through some spiritual truths that have yet to be heard. Be prepared, for some may not be ready, but it is time and you won't be alone. There are many who will get it and therefore open a whole new pathway to being in this world."

And also: "The likelihood being I [Rosa] would be released when I was ready to return to my true mission of uplifting the world and baring my soul to the masses through this kind soul who offered me her heart and her mind. Her body was not ready for me and so it is that together we began to raise our vibration so we would one day connect in the realm of spirit and she would channel my words and my life to lift you all with the truths of the cosmos."

I should have at least suspected the hugeness of the book in terms of the spiritual perspectives Rosa was sharing, but I only interpreted the words at the level I was at. Each time I've 'upgraded', I've seen more depth in them. Certainly, reading the messages below requires depth; they're fabulous, and require us to stretch our minds, hearts, and imaginations. So, if you're drawn to, read on, go ahead with an open heart and playful mind. Rosa's words may make sense to you now or perhaps later, if you're drawn to read them again at another point in time. Read her message again and again until you 'hear' it – or skip it until you feel ready and move on to the next messages and chapters. Or if you've read enough for now, jump straight to the conclusion. Rosa's intention is healing and uplifting us all into remembering who we are and bringing balance.

This book is really three books in one with each part complete in itself as well as a part of the whole book.

It's also taken me two years – from when I first started writing the book – for the penny to drop and to realise that of course this book and this life are all about creation! That is who we are, our essence. We are all created, creative and therefore creation; it's what we're here for – to create. We create in every moment. Whether that be your life or a new life. All of which not only affects you but also the collective.

What us courageous women and men are doing here through our challenging journeys to motherhood, to parenthood, is blatantly showing the world that something is very wrong, something is out of balance. If we are not creating and creative, this is against the natural law of who we are. The more out of balance this energy of creation is, the more out of balance we are in terms of being creative, the more the earth becomes out of balance.

## Separate or together?

The notion of biodiversity is well accepted. Put simply, all things are connected, and when there is an imbalance in one, this affects something else. Take bees, for example. In the British Isles alone, there are over 250 species of bee recorded, some species relying on only one kind of plant. The Colletes Hederae bee is totally dependent on ivy flowers. The ivy produces pollen, nectar, fruit, and shelter for dozens of species of insects at key times. This wealth of fruit and insects attracts a wide range of birds and mammals searching for food, shelter and nesting, and is of major ecological importance – yet to many, ivy is viewed as a destructive nuisance. Who is the destructive nuisance here? Certainly not the ivy, or the bees and creatures that thrive on it.

The habitats and food sources created by the floral mix will also expand the number of animals and plant life. If there are fewer bees and other pollinating insects, because we have destroyed their habitats for farming or simply to make an area look more attractive in some people's opinion, the result is less diversity of flora and fauna – a dying out of species. Ultimately, what is lost is our own human sources of sustenance for life. One species of tiny insect plays a huge role in the life of another and of ourselves.

As humans, we have radically altered the world around us without fully understanding the consequences. Diverting water sources, reclaiming land. And don't get me started on fracking! I was shown an image of how fracking feels to the earth and, metaphorically speaking, this action is akin to us being repeatedly punched in the gut. It's essentially punching holes in the solar plexus, the power centre, of Mother Earth. How would you feel if your seat of power, your sense of self that is held in this area of the gut, was repeatedly being drilled into?

We have all perhaps experienced 'fracking' on some personal level, essentially being disempowered, and all had different reactions to it. How is Mother Earth going to respond?

We can easily see, measure and monitor through science, biodiversity, the effect of one thing on another. Life creates more life. However, what is more difficult is seeing ourselves as part of it, part of nature, and even a part of each other as humans. We have been separated from nature and global biodiversity and therefore from ourselves, for thousands of years.

If you follow the theme running through this book, the increasing separation can be seen as the result of masculine energy, feeling the need to have control over life, over creation, being better than, more important than, thus creating ever more separation from life. I would argue this is mostly unconscious, except as I've been told, perhaps the 'few' whoever they were eons ago/are now even, wishing to have power over everything, ruling through fear. The dichotomy being that this energy is actually being fuelled by fear of not being better than or more important than but in fact the opposite – that of fear of being controlled and being inconsequential to life. The joys and conflicts of patriarchy!

The fear and imbalance creates a forgetfulness of the crucial role the masculine plays in creation of life through the seeding of life. This masculine energy in the gender male physical form is so different from the physical form of the feminine creator, the mother. Does this create an even greater sense of difference and separateness in the male? A question I'm going to ponder on further at some point.

In regard to the feminine, author Margaret Atwood's new book – The Testaments – looks deeply at the way women are dehumanised. She powerfully points out that when people are frightened and angry they give up their rights in favour of stability. Women have aimed for stability rather than stand up for their right to be themselves in every way. The trade-off has been survival.

We are all connected and our actions have consequences for us on individual, collective and universal levels. It's the imbalance that has created a sense of disconnection to our own sense of self, who you are.

Below is the unedited version of my conversation with Rosa and the promise of revealing some cosmic truths. I want to remind you of Rosa's comment at the end of Part 1 of this book about our general fear of there being nothing, or feeling nothing, or being seen as nothing – no-thing. She turned the perspective that being nothing is 'bad' into a positive truth. We are all nothing because we are whole and complete, whereas a thing can only be separate. We have been trained and have experienced being a thing – a separate thing – and to fear being whole and connected.

### Rosa's story of creation

I apologised for not connecting with her for a long time. I chatted generally about the book and asked her what the bigger message is for her/our book.

**Rosa**: There is a time and a place for everything, my dear child, and now is the time that we happen to be connecting again. That is a wonderful and thing and the only thing that you need to know right now.

For it is all coming together, my precious baby, it is all coming together and the words and the worlds are conspiring together in order to make this happen. My beautiful Debra, are you ready to hear my words now and are you ready and willing and able to write them and share them?

What we have been doing thus far is merely scratching the surface of what is, and what is happening right here and right now. Your words and mine will do many great things for the women who will read this book, but they will also do many great things for the world itself. Because what we are doing here, my darling Debra, is changing the world, changing how we see the world and how the world operates.

So yes, you can hear these words and, yes, you are ready to hear them. Relax, my little one, into the story you are about to be told. It is the story of creation itself, the creation of the universe and of the many worlds that are a part of it.

Do not fear these words and do not question them for I will help you to switch your mind away from them. The time for analysing is later and not for now. Sit back, and let go, and let me tell you a story of long, long ago when the winds first blew across from the east to the west and the north to the south. Great winds so powerful they blew the very universe and the cosmos together.

It is up to you what you wish to call these winds but for now, we see them as winds, great and powerful winds overseeing the very start of creation in an explosion of light that created a universe. It was a universe that had never once been seen in the lands of space above or beyond the nothingness. As those winds met, and as they collided, a new force was brought through into the world; because these winds connected in such a manner and with such force that they knew instantly that they were meant to be together.

They knew there and then that all they had been looking for, as they travelled around in the nothingness, was each other. The minute they met, a love was born that was beyond words. They wished for all and everyone to be able to feel the power of this love, to feel this power of connection, when four disparate winds collide and connect in a sanctity of marriage that is beyond your word sanctity.

For there are often no words to describe the love of this love that comes through when these four forces meet. And don't run away with me when I say four. I urge you to free your mind for now, my little one.

And so these four forces became one, became a whole and

within that whole became the beginnings of life. Because how could a whole not wish to become even more whole, ever more expansive, ever greater than the sum of all its parts?

In order to do this, they had to let go of some of their parts. These parts formed the lands and the planets that you see now in your universe and some of these parts are in other areas of your nothingness that you cannot see.

The whole became a part of the parts, apart from itself. And this was somewhat disturbing to the whole, and also disturbing to the parts of the whole. Where were they to go now and what were they to do? How was it that they would once again join together as an even greater and bigger part of the whole, a huge expanse of the love and explosion of light that had come from that very first connection?

## Planetary communication

So, the parts (planets) and the whole (Source/Grand Central Sun/Creator energy) agreed to reconvene at certain points in time and to check in on each and everyone's experience of this wholeness. But also as 'not wholeness'.

So, every now and then at certain points, there is a meeting, a convening of these planets, and they give and share and swap their stories and their insights into what it means to be a whole, but also a part of the [original] whole.

Do you see my dear, how, when you read your planets in your sky, what it is that they are doing? And know also that the same thing is happening in other areas of the whole that you cannot see.

So to continue my story, as each and every planet wished to learn and to grow in its nature and its stature, it took on certain personalities as you would see it. And each personality grew stronger and stronger until they became so strong they too had no choice but to separate some of their wholeness into parts in order for them also to see what it was like to be whole but separate. To look back at themselves through these parts.

And these are the parts that you are seeing today. The parts that have grown from a molecule or a star and the parts that have grown from the earth and the sky. All these parts are essentially a big part of the whole of the four winds, but also a part of the whole of their own part. Third generation parts of the whole if you like.

This is not something to be getting your head around quite yet, as we are speaking. So do not try to figure it all out as you are writing, my dear, and simply keep on writing my words as you are hear them, for hearing them you are my love, my channel, my light, my part. Do you see the depth of the message we had for each other when I said to you my 'unwholeness' in your human eyes led to you becoming whole? And at the same time led to me becoming whole? Because we were together and then we were apart and yet always one.

And this is why you can hear me, my dear, because we are of that One. And this is why others can hear other parts of themselves, because they too are One. But I am digressing. I will you to sit back and to switch off your racing mind and to listen to the rest of my tale.

As each of the planets grew and merged and grew again and separated again, each and every one of them swapped information and consciousness about their experience as a whole part, of a part of the whole.

Within each of these parts of the whole, still more parts were conceived in ways that will blow your mind. For some were conceived of vessels and some were conceived of light. Some were conceived from the merging of the planets and some were conceived of the earth. This is the part that you will most likely understand, my dear, for the earth is just one part of a very big whole. The wholeness of the love that was created at the merging, the connection, and the explosion of the four winds.

## We are One

Who or what are these four winds, I hear you ask? In your terms, my dear, you would classify these four winds as the hearts and the minds, the bodies and the souls of the human. But in reality, the four winds were of the nothingness that was nothing until, by chance, one day, they met, they collided and they became as one. Just as it is with humans and just as it is with all the beings on your planet and beyond.

For each and every one of you and each and every one of them is made up from the wholeness that came from the joining of those four parts.

Do you see, my dear, that as you humans are made up of these four winds, these four parts, then so too is everyone and everything on your planet. And not only that, but every planet and each and every being on their planets. We are of the whole, they are of the whole, the planets are of the whole and the only difference is in the way we experience the whole.

And that, my dear, is a great lesson for your humanity, because you are always judging. You are always minding and mithering about who is who and what is what and who has and who has not. The lesson is that each and every one of you has it all and is the all – the all and everything of the all.

Therefore, it is not a surprise that life can get confusing sometimes. That in each and everyone's desperation to scramble back to that first place of wholeness, that first place of love, and to experience that sense of the explosion of love, you can find yourself scrambling over others to get there, not realising you are actually scrambling and treading on yourself.

And so, my dear, that is the story of the universe and a very small story at that for this story is written for you from the human perspective. As it is written and experienced on other planets, and by other beings, the details will be very much the same and yet different.

Because, just as you are all the same, you are all very different. And just as a planet is a planet made up from the four forces of the universe, so it is that they too are different. Each and every one of you brings something different and unique to the table, so too do each and every planet and each and every being and force on these planets.

You can see the planets merging and changing as they swap information. From your earthly point of view they are doing this for you and it is most certainly having an effect on you, for you all feel that you are the centre of your own universes.

Yet, do you see that the merging and the moving of the planets will have similar or different effects on the evolution and the beings of those other planets – some of whom still think, and some of whom are more advanced than to think, that they are the centre of the universe? With the truth, of course, being that you are all at the centre of the universe because you are the universe.

You are the four pieces of the puzzle that were conceived and created as the universe you now know and the universe that you don't yet know.

And so, my dear, how does this story sit with you? I am ready to move on as I know you are waiting for me to get to the crux of the story that involves you and me and the story that on your own planet, Earth, has played out for so long. The story of the birth of the Mother itself, the Mother Earth.

## Portals of travel and creation

As with all the planets, Earth was created from the part of

the whole that held this consciousness of love at its highest form. There is no reason for this as such. It is just how it was decided. And so many beings wished to be a part of this consciousness and a part of this earth. Indeed, many beings often travelled there or lived there and even chose to remain there, mixing with the other beings from that planet.

Some of these were creatures and some of these were simply energy. All they had in common was the breath of life that came from the I am of the I am, the God-consciousness, the love of the four winds of consciousness.

Yet, they lived in peace and they explored the land and each other and they also explored the skies and the stars and they travelled between them as they so wished. For they all knew that they were of the universe and not only of the planet Earth.

As they zipped around the cosmos as and when they pleased, the knowledge they shared and the knowledge they gained helped to grow and expand the very nature of the cosmos, and indeed the very nature of the I am presence – the whole.

Days went by and love filled the land as this knowledge was exchanged and shared, given and received by all of those who happened across it. This was not a time of secrets; it was a time of love.

It was a time of expansion and harmony. As this knowledge and this love were shared, this information became closer to the light of knowledge, the light of truth, the light of Source, and the light of the four winds of consciousness, in order for these parts and this part of the Universe to once again converge and re-join the wholeness and oneness of the God-consciousness, as you call it.

Then the Earth itself exploded in an abundance of this love and beauty in the form of flowers and more and varied creatures, each one yet again a part of the all-encompassing Whole.

This was a time of great beauty and a time of great flourishing for the Earth and its people, and its beings of light who had settled there, and its creatures. And the Earth was so close to the heart of God and to returning to the heart of God as a Whole that, for some, this was too much to bear.

## Corruption and the fall of Oneness

They could not bear the light of the Earth, and they could not stomach the intensity and the light of the Earth, for they had not experienced the birth of the Earth. They were the newcomers and the explorers and the ones setting out on their own adventures of the planets, only to find that once they reached Earth, they found themselves wanting. They felt disgruntled that they had missed out and been cheated of the opportunity of growing up on this planet.

Their mission was to take a hold of your planet and to take a hold of the love that they themselves couldn't bear. And they all wished to have and to take what they wanted from Earth and carry it back to their own planets.

They didn't get that there was nothing to take, for it was all given. And everything they ever wanted was here for them to share and be shared. And yet this is not what happened, and so our tale begins.

For as these beings began to integrate and to ingratiate themselves into the lives of the planet Earth and all its beings. They began to shift and move the energy from one of abundance and one of love, to one of fear and one of lack.

Slowly, ever so slowly, the weak and the vulnerable were convinced of their unworthiness, convinced of their role as the lame, the sick, the unwanted, and tolerated and yet not as loved as the loved ones. And so it was that eventually the tables were turned and the balance was shifted from one of love and compassion, one of sharing of the knowledge that was held in and of the Earth, to one of the corruption of the Earth.

I experienced an overwhelming tiredness and also guilt that felt like boredom! I was feeling guilty. I wasn't as excited as I should be about all this information as I was wondering: how on earth does this fit in with the book? Looking back, maybe it wasn't boredom but sheer overwhelm at the power of Rosa's energy coming through me, and my human mind trying to make sense of it all. Maybe I was re-living the soul trauma as consciousness began to shift and move to an unknown place. Trauma can make us want to pass out, go to sleep, as our conscious minds can't comprehend what is happening. Maybe you're in the same place as I was then reading it. Go with whatever it is you're feeling.

At the time, I felt my ego-mind had jumped in and I felt almost like a child having a tantrum when I said: what has all this got to do with our book?! I said as much and reconnected with Rosa whose reply was, "But as with all of life, until you understand the root of that life or the root of that pain, then how will you ever alter that root to change and to grow and see it to pluck it out altogether if that's what needs to happen? This will be the basis for so much more than your book."

**Rosa continues**

> And so Earth fell and the love and the knowledge fell into the deepest, darkest heart of itself in order to keep itself safe.

> As we see ourselves reflected in the Earth, the heart of the knowledge, wisdom, and power, which is of course the power of Divine Love, it is kept held within and locked away in the beautiful consciousness and heart of Mother Earth herself.

> For the wounds here are deep and you could say that this was the original wound of the mother. A wound that came when her giving and her trust, her openness and her heart, were literally on show for all to receive in offer for the greater good of the expansion of the whole universe – the whole, the all and everything of the all and everything, of which she, Mother Earth, was a part. A part that contained and gave so much love, it was so very close to once again joining with the Whole from which she had come. And yet she suffered

for her openness, she suffered for her light shining so brightly, attracting all and everyone to it. She suffered for her abundance and her creations and her life-giving force, and she suffered for standing out as the one who was closest to God out of all the planets.

For what those planets, or at least many beings from those planets didn't realise, was that they too were as close to God, but as a part of the 'Whole' of God that was experiencing this wholeness in their own unique way.

Never above or below, never more right or wrong, and never closer or further apart, but simply different. A different whole of the whole but still a 'whole' part, a holy part of the grand I AM.

And as I can see you thinking, my dear, yes, you can see how this story has played out in your world many, many, many times. As if the Earth is calling you, beckoning you to remember the love that once shone here and so brightly it was considered the heart of the cosmos. And you can see it in your readings and you can see it in your teachings.

## You are the Universe

So, dear Debra, when you were wondering 'where on earth' I was going with this story, and what it had to do with your story, do you see, my dear, that it is indeed the all and everything of your story? Because if the all and everything of the Whole is the all and everything of the planets, and if the all and everything of the planets is the all and everything of the beings, and creative life forces on those planets, then you are all indeed the planets playing the parts of that whole. And these planets are playing the parts of the 'Whole' of all that is.

And so as your planets, do you see which of your human stories have been playing out this original story? This original wound of the mother? And that mother being Mother Earth?

And if all of your stories and your legends are merely whole parts, of the greater whole, then can you see how, if each whole part heals the wounds of the mother of the mother of the mother, and of all mothers, it will eventually be that the very great Earth Mother, the Mother of all earth mothers, will be able to rise once again?

Once more be able to shine, to love, to create, and be able to be with God. Be able and free to share once again her secrets and her knowledge, and once again become the life force of the universe of all universes.

Do you see how great your work is? And do you see how great and magnificent the work is of all of you lightworkers who have chosen to come to Earth, or rise up from the Earth once again in order to show the Earth that it is indeed time for her to reveal her full and whole self to the cosmos once again?

For just as you know, and very many women on your planet know, there is so much more depth to their being than they currently show. There is so much more wisdom, more love, more nurturing, abundance, and creativity that lies within them – just as it is at the heart of our Mother of all mothers: our Mother Earth.

And so we will begin to unpick the stories of your lands for which this story has played out over millennia.

Phew! To bring this message back to you the individual, which is easier for us all to understand, basic physics tells us we are all energy – everything is energy. We can look at your body and how it operates. Science knows and shows that every one of the trillions of your tiny cells in your body is a whole universe in and of itself. Each of your cells is constantly shifting and moving and communicating with its environment, experiencing itself as a whole part of a bigger whole; co-creating experiences, physical and emotional, with the rest of its whole, your body – and the rest of the universe – its environment.

Rosa's message just expands that concept, highlighting for me, at least, the message that we are not separate from anything but 'a part' of it all. For more discussion on the science of cellular biology and how each cell and each person interacts with the environment, and their environment – including that of the body, the mind, and external environments – I highly recommend the work of Dr Bruce Lipton. There are so many highly qualified women and men of science who offer scientific explanations, if you are interested in this aspect. These include Dr Kelly Brogan, Gregg Braden, Dr Christiane Northrup, and Dr Joe Dispenza, to name a few. You'll find the ones on YouTube and the Internet that you're drawn to personally.

Khalil Gibran brings this concept of Oneness in within his text, 'The Eye of the Prophet', with his thought that all of creation exists within you. Also that everything that exists within you, is also in creation. So basically, what you feel on the inside, you'll see in your outside world. If you're seeing it, you're creating it. If you don't like what you see, go within and transform how you feel about what you're seeing.

## Decoding the Universe

There are many ways we've found for decoding the universe. I've never been big on maths so I can't talk about mathematical patterns. But for those of you who have the aptitude, you may want to check out the many formulas and theories that maths provides to understand the patterns of our universe – the Fibonacci sequence, for example.

Our ancient ancestors, who only had the earth and the stars to work with, were genius at figuring out the patterns of the universe. The pyramids, Stonehenge, New Grange, Machu Picchu, were all incredible feats of engineering using mathematical concepts – nothing at all primitive as we like to view previous civilisations and communities. They also all align with planetary movements.

The science of numerology I am far more at home with, and it is another way we try and decipher the world. The number 4 holds huge spiritual significance. It has been described as the number of 'being', the number that connects mind, body, and spirit with the physical world of structure and organisation. It symbolises the safety and security of 'home.' It's the number of justice and stability and, in Soul plan Readings, the 4 holds the energy of fertility and abundance. The spiritual nature of 4 is creating a sacred space and sanctuary. In the Bible, number 4 is associated with the creation of the world. Think of the four seasons, the four elements, the four directions of north, south, east, and west. When Rosa said the universe was formed from the meeting of the four 'winds' – I can see why this number holds so much meaning spiritually. It is the energy of creation.

As with all life, there is polarity and it's the same with numbers. The opposite of creation is destruction. In Soul plan I mentioned that the 4 is the energy of abundance and fertility. Its challenging aspects are: mistrust, feeling abandoned, isolation, feeling unworthy of and being unable to create. Are we living more in the challenging aspect of this 4 energy of creation rather than being in balance and living and embodying the essence of creation?

The importance of restoring balance through healing our wounds as women and men, saying yes to ourselves as powerful, magical, creative, sovereign beings, allowing the Divine Mother energy to rise, be seen, acknowledged and felt, cannot be understated. As Rosa said in her message about the New Earth at the start of this book, the New Earth is essentially the old earth, the original earth that was one of unity and unconditional love, open to all. The shifting energies, however dramatic and challenging they may appear at times, are helping us all to remember our original state of being, our return to unity and love.

The following message from Rosa is huge. I know I say they're all huge but this one threw me for quite a while. I even contemplated not putting it in here at all, but then right now I don't know where else to share it and it needs to be heard.

I didn't ask for this message, I was actually connecting with Rosa to ask her about egg donation and this is what she wanted to share with me instead. This message is why I say the power and importance of you cannot be underestimated. To stand in love and shine this out. To recognise the wounds and heal them.

At the time of writing this book, every day you'd hear news about the destruction of the planet, and the plundering of her resources. And, in the United Kingdom, the ever-increasing private property rules that see only a few benefit from the expanse of nature, land and rivers included; and the building of the HS2 railway line running from South to North of England that has desecrated ancient woodlands, once heralded for their beauty and significance. Why is all this happening?

The destruction of Mother Earth is the destruction of the mother. Without the mother, there is no more life. This isn't just about the Earth, it's about women. If looking after the Earth and being in union with her seems too intangible and far away to contemplate, then think of a world without women who can no longer create. Without women in their magnificent, powerful, creative selves, Earth or not, there is no more life.

If we as women continue to give away our power, stay separate from other women because of old wounds such as jealousy and betrayal, do not support men with their healing and expressing their feminine side, essentially not address the mother wound, the imbalance may slide further along the scale towards destruction rather than creation. I know this sounds like a bad movie. When I was telling my husband about Rosa's message, he had the expression of 'right, how do I deal with this one and not say the wrong thing even though I have no idea what she's talking about'! And then he said: isn't there a film like that called Children of Men with Clive Owen. Genius. We then had to watch the film, which isn't a bad movie at all.

I did go into fear with this message (and the film). However, as my super gifted friend Sarah Impey says, it's all about going into the fear, into the dark, because it's in there where your power lies. Sarah is working on her own channelling and theories about the energy of the 666 number – a number we've all been led to fear. However, her findings are that this is a Divine feminine number; again, we've been focusing on the negative polarity of this number to fear it when it is actually where we come into our power. I feel there will be more of this type of turning old beliefs and fears on their head, coming from all aspects and angles, so we can 'see' more clearly where the veils have been pulled down over our eyes.

We've been taught to fear, feeling fearful. However, if we embrace fear, explore it, go into our own dark, we find our Divine feminine, we find ourselves more free than ever before, because there's no longer anything to fear. We find our power. So I did. And I realised that the course of destruction it can look like we're on, is a possible timeline, but there are so many other potential timelines. We, each and every one of us, have a choice in which timeline we hop onto. We're powerful beings of light, limitless in what we're capable of.

As I moved through the panic, I remembered my Aboriginal guide showing me a New Dawn and the feeling of joy and peace that came with it. I remembered all the spirit babies, their energy of unconditional love, their wisdom, plans and playfulness, and their messages of arriving to help bring about this New Dawn, the New Earth. I was asked in 2020 if it was responsible to bring a child into the world at this time. When I asked Rosa, she said, it's the exact right time to bring new life and welcome new souls into the world because they are needed to bring about the new.

There is a higher plan, one which we may not see or even grasp, but if we do our bit, they'll do theirs. I also remembered the overwhelming and indescribable beauty of feeling unconditional love from the Divine Mothers, the galactics, and other light beings. This energy is in the world, and if this energy is in the world for us all to access, then we really are going to be okay. It's so much more powerful than fear, it has no agenda, it just is. We are all this unconditional love; it's just been a little bit buried under stuff. I've seen the New Earth, felt it, it's creation and not destruction we're heading to. And you, incredible women, are part of it. Go into your fears, go into your dark knowing you are so held in love, emerging as the shimmering light of joy you are, fully in your natural creation, creative being.

# Rosa on the energy of the Mother

This information came through when I was in meditation with psychic artist and gifted healer Jenny Parris, and Archangels Michael, Jophiel, and Raphael, when I saw in my earth star chakra (the chakra that lies about 15 inches in the earth below your feet and is your unique connection point with Mother Earth) a trunk that was filled with stuff, much of which I no longer needed. I was encouraged to dig deeper and see what was in it. I then saw a sceptre; somehow I knew it was the sceptre of Mother Mary. I carried this throughout my meditation, through all the chakras in curiosity. (I still haven't quite figured out what I'm meant to do with the sceptre but I'm sure it will become clear at some point!)

I then needed to ask Rosa about the energy of egg donation for the egg donor. What came through instead was this message.

**Rosa on the energy of the Mother**

> You take up the mantle of love of Mary, do you know what this means? You become a representative of all mothers, you become a voice of all mothers and you become all mothers.
>
> Do you know what this means my love, my heart? You must do your work with even greater focus. The work of Mary is the work of God; the work of God is the work of the Universe and the work of the Universe is the work of life itself, all life.
>
> Without the mother, there can be no more life. Do you see what is happening here, my dear? They are trying to replace the mother. They are trying to destroy their own selves because that is the pattern they are in, the experience they are in, of always needing to attack the mother because they cannot bear to look at themselves – and therefore they hate the mother for bringing them into existence.
>
> They blame the mother, they cannot bear the mother because the mother is a reflection of their own wants and needs and they cannot find it within themselves and they cannot find it within the mother. And so the mother is to

blame for them finding themselves in this predicament.

It is of the utmost importance to protect the mothers at this time as they are in need of much help. A great battle they are fighting for their very existence. It is the energy of the mother that can birth all and give all and yet it is not happening in this way as yet, as mothers do not understand the very key concept that they are life.

They are life, they are the life, the life of the whole universe and you will return to the nothingness of the All before the 'big bang', before the explosion of light. And there will be nothing. Not the nothing that is 'no thing', the whole, the all – but nothing – nothing at all.

There will be no existence. And the ones who hurt and the ones who harm the mother are the very ones who need the help to see that it is not the mother that is to blame for their ills but their twisted sense of self and lack of recognition of the light they are. For they only live in the dark and can only see the dark and so therefore the lens they are viewing the world with is purely the dark, there is no light.

The damage is such that nothing can be done about those who are in this state of being. However, there is plenty to be done for those who are not.

And it is those who do not, who must be the ones who shine up and shine up so brightly that the dark can only live in the dark and not bring its darkness into the world. It is held at bay, it is seen and helped and loved and yet has no light to control or manipulate and attempt to take from the mother and destroy the mother.

The more mothers you help in this way to know only of the light and not only just of the dark and the need to destroy the mother for all the pain she has brought, when they (the holders of the consciousness of control and fear) realise that they are the ones in pain and realise that they are the ones who destroy, not the mother, not God, not the universe, but they.

And when they reach this point of understanding – that it is only the light, the love and the power of the mother who can hold this dark in unconditional love – then they will be and see the very existence of the universe itself.

And so it is.

The image I saw as this message was coming through was that of the whole world and billions of lights covering the planet. There was a tiny corner of the world that was still dark but because of the sheer amount of light, each and every point of light, this dark could be there, could be loved and acknowledged but it held no power whatsoever.

The image reminded me of Rosa's message at the end of Part 1 that stated maybe we and our children might want to 'play' in the darker fields of consciousness every now and again to remember or to learn, but it will be a thing of the past that we'll be living in these darker or lower energies on a daily basis. Those energies of guilt, blame, shame, distorted power and division, to name a few. The more we choose to play about in the fields of joy and cooperation, because we do have a choice, and the more we choose to acknowledge, heal and release the lower energies, the more likely this image of a world full of light and a little bit of dark will be seen and felt by us all – and most certainly our children and their children.

You can do this, you absolutely have this. Peel back the layers, lift the veil and be curious as to who you are, not who you have been taught to be.


## More signs from the Universe


Astronomy and astrology are revealing more and more about the creation of our universe. Rosa paints a scene of cosmic travel with beings from all over the universe zipping about wherever they wish to go. I do this most days sitting in my lounge and connecting in with either my own or my clients' soul histories – it's fascinating! Think of the films Star Wars or Star Trek – any sci-fi movie or book – and it feels they are not so far from the truth. I read an article from a physicist recently that was entitled: 'Science proves portals are real'. A dramatic headline for sure but there are definitely ongoing studies around portals and NASA has apparently found electron markers to locate and study them.

One of my boys' favourite films at the moment is 'The Kid who would be King' – a modern-day take on the legend of King Arthur. They travel through a portal at Stonehenge to Cornwall and near to Merlin's Cave. This stuff is becoming mainstream and enabling more and more people to open up to the bigger picture of who they are, where they fit in the grand scheme of things and what's possible.

The legend of King Arthur may well be one of the legends Rosa refers to as 'playing out the story of the universe'. Perhaps my next book will be relating our myths, legends and stories to the story of creation and how it was corrupted. In the King Arthur story, for example, King Arthur's half-sister Morgana or Morgan Le Fay, is depicted in many ways and as time goes on, particularly from the middle ages, she moves from being an otherworldly fairy healer to being terrifying and downright wrong – using her witchy powers to bring about the downfall of man. Does this theme ring any bells? Powerful, magical woman equals evil. I look forward to the true Morgana story coming to light.

The story of the search for the Holy Grail is one that intrigues me. In a meditation, again in my Divine Mother Meditation Group, we were guided by Goddess Isis into the Holy Grail itself. The Holy Grail was revealed as the wombs of the women. The secrets and deep wisdom held in the womb. This meditation was for women and there is no reason it's not the same for men, after all, at some point in time the majority of us have lived as both genders and men have energetic wombs – although not many like to hear this! We all hold the masculine and feminine energy and therefore all of us hold the wisdom. I believe the story of the search for the Holy Grail is a story representing the search for ourselves, our truth, as the explosion of love we all are.

Whilst we're here talking about wombs and questioning the various stories we're told about certain characters, let's look at the word 'whore'. The earth child that is Lucy Hodgens researched and shared this information about the word whore, harlot and others that are derogatory to women. It's fascinating and again helps us to reframe what we grow up with and are conditioned to feel and know. If anyone is to create a book turning history and the myths and legends upside down to another perspective, it's Lucy.

This is what she discovered. The great womb of creation, the pre-existent birther of All, was once known as the Great Whore. In the sematic languages of the Middle East, hor meant "cave" or "womb". She was also known as a harlot – a "womb of light".

In Hebrew, the word horaa meant "instruction" and the word hor meant "Light". It was from these holy hor root words that the Torah, the Old Testament, took its name. The Womb of Light was always known as the lawgiver, the teacher, the enlightener, the light bearer. Horasis was the ancient Greek word for Womb Enlightenment, bestowed through the sexual union of man and woman. In the Bible, horasis was used to describe an oracular, ecstatic vision. Horus in Egyptian mythology is the Divine Child of Goddess Isis and is known for his ability to travel between worlds. He helps us to access our psychic insights, wisdom and light.

Throughout the world, we discover these feminine womb words at the foundation of spiritual worship, root words such as her, har, hor, hera, hara, and hero. In ancient Babylon, Ishtar was called the Great Goddess Har, Mother of Harlots. Her high priestess, the Harine, was considered the spiritual ruler of the city of Ishtar.

In the indigenous Huichol tradition of Mexico, the name for the primordial grandmother Goddess of the ocean is Haramara: Womb of Mother.

These root words are also found, sequestered like magical pearls, inside words such as chariot, chorus, charm, and harmony. Harmony literally means "to be in tune with the moon or womb cycles". The word charis is the name that the Holy men of India, devotees of Shiva/Shakti, give to the entheogens they smoke. It means "Goddess" or "Menstrual Blood", and is also the root word of the Christian word eucharist.

It is time to remember and reclaim the beauty and sanctity of our inner whore, our inner harlot, our Great Womb of Light – the original Holy Feminine.

## The signs are everywhere

In every kids' film I watch I see a deeper meaning and a pattern, a reflection of the universe. It drives my husband bonkers. Kids' films such as Coco – with its messages of life and love after death – and Frozen 2 –how we can change our realities by opening up that memory file, accessing the energy, emotions and decisions we made at that time, and supporting our earlier selves, or our ancestors, to transform them in the matrix. Also, The Black Panther and other Marvel films, with their tales of other beings and realms. Who says other realms don't exist? In Part 1 of this book we travelled to the spirit baby realm. Just because we can't see something doesn't mean it doesn't exist.

Before I became a mum I had no idea what that mum world had to offer. After 10am the streets, parks and community centres were filled with mums and babies and they'd all but disappeared by 5pm when the workers were on their way home. It felt like another world within a world that I hadn't been aware of until I needed to be. I knew nothing about the motorsport speedway, had never even heard of it before I met my husband. I had no idea it existed. But it does and takes up quite a lot of my world now!

## Which part of the story are you playing out?

How many worlds are out there in the world that you don't know about? Just because they are not in your awareness doesn't mean they don't exist; they just don't exist for you. I see the universe in the same way. Once we see it and experience it, it exists. And we can absolutely travel to anywhere within it when we go deep into ourselves. All of our answers are within us. The reason we have an opportunity to find our answers and go zipping about the universe in our minds is because each of us is the universe. You are of the same energy and so can communicate with the energy.

You are a whole part of another part, which is a whole part of another part, and so on and so on until you reach right back to the original planets and the original energy of creation, the four winds as Rosa describes it, the big bang.

In a nutshell, how I read this is that having been created and being a creator: we are all creation. You are born of and with the energy of creation and therefore your purpose here is to create and to experience yourself further through your creations, whether that be life experiences, physical creations, or new life. You are born of the ability to create, to manifest. You as a woman are a whole part of something bigger. You as a man are a whole part of something bigger. Your baby is a whole part of you, the whole woman and the whole man, and a whole part of something bigger. We are all parts of a greater whole going back and back to the original whole – the four winds, the big bang, the creation of the Universe. And we as energy in form are recreating this story of creation time and time again.

What story of the universe and of creation are you playing out? Does this mean that if we become aware of our stories and the timelines we're living, we can change or drop those stories and timelines until we are all playing out the one timeline of the explosion of love, the timeline to feeling whole and 'home' within ourselves?

## Imbalance in creation

The second part of this creation story as told by Rosa above, addresses the distortion of the creation energy, which is the imbalance of the masculine and feminine energies that occurred when those who didn't like what they saw, began to control and corrupt. Masculine creation energy began to control, with the aim of having power over the female aspect of creation. This was driven by a sense of being separate and different from the energies of the earth, the mother, and led to fear of being inconsequential, not as powerful, and also the fear of lack – the fear of not having and owning all the energy of creation.

In short, it is this imbalance that we see every day in our physical lives. This is seen as war – over land, people, religion, resources – due to this intense, ancient fear of lack, of not owning the power to create, so having to take it, or alternatively, having to settle for less. The distortion in the energy of creation is creating war, and more lack and fear rather than love. We all create from either a place of fear or from a place of love. Are you reacting out of fear or out of love? That's a question we all need to ask ourselves in regard to the choices we make.

We also see it with greed and in those who feel the need to accumulate and hold onto more and more resources – the Scrooge energy. Is it that those who have control over lots of resources without the pure philanthropic aspect of giving back to balance it, deep down and unconsciously know they have 'taken', from the earth or people, what they do not own? Is it the fear that they risk losing it all and losing control again?

It also plays out in struggling to conceive because we have been forced and/or have chosen to give away our creative power. We are continually creating and recreating the story of this imbalance. Absorbing often harsh lessons and wounds in our ability or inability to create. When hurt and pain pushes deep into ourselves, we have little choice but to scrutinise the pain and the personal 'why'; to remember our creative power and right to create and restore balance in order to heal our individual wounds, in turn healing the collective and universal wounds.

# Adoption and how it plays a part in healing the universe

Adoption is another way in which we play out the story of creation. I originally intended to add a section on adoption in Chapter 7: The many ways of coming into the world. However, Rosa's message on adoption felt too big to fit there. I was even going to leave it out altogether because there is much more to explain and explore than I currently have the knowledge and information for right now. There is no question, however, that adoption is extremely challenging and complex for everyone involved.

In Robert Schwartz's book, 'Your Soul's Plan: Discovering the Real Meaning of the Life You Planned Before You Were Born', adoption is a soul's choice. A soul choice of the birth mother, the child, and the adoptive parents. As you've read in this book, each and every one of us made choices about what we wish to experience in this lifetime. Robert Schwartz writes about the contracts made between souls to ensure the child soul is conceived through the birth mother – offering the gift of life – and then another contract is made with the foster parents and/or adoptive parents – offering the gift of support and guidance, or more lessons. Each party agrees to the terms of these contracts. (These contracts can be renegotiated.) Walter Makichen, in his book, 'Spirit Babies: How to communicate with the child you're meant to have', asserts that – one way or another – the soul will find its way to its intended parents. You are destined to be together and will find each other. I would recommend both books for their discussion on adoption and many other aspects of life and soul choices.

I expected a similar message from Rosa when I asked her why a soul would choose adoption. I also asked her how we can best serve those who make this choice to help them understand it and themselves better. I should know by now not to have any expectations on Rosa's answers. Rosa being Rosa takes the discussion to another level altogether. This is why I've included it here in Part 3 and the bigger, bigger picture of the universe and the role we each play.

The extreme nature of the separation from the mother felt by those who are adopted most often leads them to a very deep sense of not feeling good enough and unworthiness. Not to mention trauma and threat to life around the uncertainty of whether they are wanted during their time in the womb. I've had the absolute pleasure of doing a soul plan reading for one gorgeous soul who was adopted and who had nothing but love and gratitude for both her birth mother – as the one to allow her to arrive in the world – and her adopted parents – who gave her the opportunity to grow. Her soul plan energies were extremely high vibration, unity consciousness, and her soul mission was to see and help others to see the beauty in all things, the positive, light side of a situation. She said on some level she'd always known it was her choice to experience this.

Most often, however, the trauma of this separation is immense, no matter how many days into life this happens. When I read the energy of children and adults who are adopted, I often see their energy body outside of their physical bodies. We all know the saying 'I jumped out of my skin' when something unexpected happens. Big traumas can leave us frozen in time, not fully in our bodies because it's not safe to be embodied. People who have been adopted may feel it's not safe to be on the earth and may find many ways to distract and distance themselves from this because they are trying to protect themselves from feeling the intense emotions surrounding separation.

In adulthood, this may lead to addictive patterns of behaviour. Many children are labelled with behaviour problems when I believe they are actually re-living their separation trauma time and time again and find it hard to stay grounded and present. They simply don't feel safe. This is the same for anyone who has experienced a traumatic birth and not just adoption. Heal your birth and the birth of your babies and your life and theirs will transform. Feeling safe in our bodies and on earth is key to us thriving. Connecting with nature and running around barefoot is a good place to start.

Birth parents, foster parents, and adoptive parents all need huge amounts of support, zero judgement, and ways to identify and move through their own patterns, beliefs, and traumas that will inevitably be triggered by their children, who, as with all children, come in as our teachers.

Only the bravest, oldest souls are willing to take on this role, with many lessons and potential healing of all aspects of this separation wound for the birth parents and those who choose the route as their foster or adopted parents, whether in loving or challenging relationships.

Babies, as we know, are conscious beings from before conception and receive and communicate just as any living being. Rosa's message on adoption will, I hope, help all those recognise the hugeness of their task on a universal scale. They are the opposite of not good enough. The service they offer the world, particularly if they choose to, and are able to find ways through the intense emotions surrounding separation, transforms the energy of separation we all feel to some degree. It works for their own benefit and for us all. They are pure service souls with immense power. Their purpose is to highlight the energy of separation, for themselves, their families, the collective, and the universe. At its ultimate conclusion, those who choose the route of adoption are playing out the timeline of the separation of the planets from Source and down the line as the planets created more parts of themselves, including us.

Those who are living the adoption timeline also highlight the wounds of the mother, the wounds of the Divine Feminine. This plays out whether giving up her child or not being able to conceive. There are many and varying beliefs and opinions around adoption. Now you know they are high souls healing ancient wounds, has it changed your opinion?

Below is the snippet from Rosa's story of creation that I believe is the timeline and the energy that adoption is playing out. The deepest wound of all is separation from their Source of life, in this case, the mother.

> In order to do this, they [the four winds of creation/Source] had to let go of some of their parts. These parts formed the lands and the planets that you see now in your universe and some of these parts are in other areas of your nothingness that you cannot see.

The whole [Source] became apart from itself. And this was somewhat disturbing to the whole, and also disturbing to the parts of the whole. Where were they to go now and what were they to do? How was it that they would once again join together as an even greater and bigger part of the whole, a huge expanse of the love and explosion of light that had come from that very first connection?

*Schwartz and Makichen* talk about contracts, in Rosa's message below she uses the term 'lines of communication'.

### Rosa on Adoption. How can we heal the wound of being given away?

Adoption is not an easy thing to understand and it is not an easy thing to experience. It is with the utmost love that I share this message for all you women and all you mums who have been at the mercy of, and yet again had some option to go with, or not, this line of mothering, of family, of finding space on this earth.

There are very many lines of communication that come before a soul is eventually birthed onto your planet and therefore just as many infinite possibilities of the ways those lines of communication play out.

So maybe one line of communication would be to simply be birthed upon the earth but choose to be birthed in a different location to the family you would choose to spend much of your time.

Or perhaps there is another line of communication that becomes open to you and that is the line of non-importance, non-citizenship, non-identity. By being given, in order to be taken away, is something the soul wishes to experience in order to repair some previous damage that has occurred between the partnership of this soul and its birth parents.

There is the line of communication by another who has previously done you harm in a past lifetime, in order to make up for the harm in this lifetime. The anger that surrounds this is tenfold from the harm you too once received in a previous life and may now give back in the form of revenge. Until you release and realise there is no such thing as revenge. It is simply a pain for your own self to be able to fill and heal at the behest of those parents who, in this lifetime, wish to help and guide you on your way to filling it.

Do you see the complications that abound from this experience you call adoption? For it is not an adoption of a person, it is an adoption of the pain of the soul who has chosen this time to come in to heal the pain that is already present. It will take an awful lot of love and an awful lot of self-awareness in order for this pain to be healed. But when it is, the power of 'no more pain' is so incredibly profound it is difficult to put into words the extreme nature of the healing that comes from this. I will attempt to explain it.

## The bigger picture – Healing Separation

What we are talking about here is the deep wound of the mother and the mother of all mothers – Mother Earth. The mother of all mothers who has come into our lives as the planet of love. So often this planet has been hurt, abused, and rejected. The storms that have attempted to take the mother out of the mother, take the mother heart out of the mother, are profound. Yet they are also few and far between despite the perception otherwise.

So deep is this wound, it appears to be at the very core of the existence of the planet, that this Source love, this mother love and abundance is about to be taken away at any moment. Therefore it is hard to trust the mother to keep you safe. You also find it hard to trust yourselves with the mother, for it is the mother who has let you down by separating herself from Source and from you. The mother has also been the cause of your greatest sense of shame – as in some lifetimes you, too, have found yourself abusing the mother for what you could get out of her.

You, my dear ones, are the product of this, the children of this. You are here to play out this story of the birth of the universe until all aspects of these possible lines of communication between the heavens and the earth are lived and experienced. All infinite potentials are played out to the very end of time in order for the two to come wholly together once more.

What has this to do with adoption, I hear you cry? Well, do you see how the father gave the seed and the mother grew the seed but there were no lines of infinite potential, there was only one? And that one was for the two not to meet in creation, but to meet in separation of self and in separation of God and in separation of the mother.

What is one meant to do with this information: the sense of aloneness, of belonging to no one and no thing? Surely that person must start to belong entirely to themselves? To rely on themselves, see themselves as their own infinite lines of potential, and for their separated selves to become their own whole creators?

And so, they become the whole once again, for they have taken themselves out and put themselves back into a position of starting afresh, starting anew from a position of wholeness and not a position of brokenness – as the soul has surely come in to heal this sense of brokenness.

Yet this has not and will not answer your question about how to heal this aspect of oneself. It is up to the individual to heal themselves, to understand their own game and their role in this game of life.

They can begin by starting to see this experience as a healing of the whole from the separation – and the cycles this may bring. Then maybe they will understand the cycles more fully and therefore understand themselves more fully.

This does not only affect the individual but also the collective, as all of those involved in the process begin to come to their own understanding of separation within the whole that is being whole, even when separate.

This is very hard to understand, and difficult to come to terms with in one lifetime. Yes, they should know that they do have many more lifetimes to come to this conclusion, if they so choose. Nothing is being forced here. These souls are honoured for any sense of wholeness they bring to the world amid their experience of separateness.

Now to the connector necessary for this to happen, for who do they connect with? For all souls are connected and therefore need to find their connector. Could it be that they are able to reconnect with those very souls who gave them away in the first place? That it is this service of understanding and forgiveness that can bring about the sense of wholeness and connection that they so crave – connection without the trauma of disconnection.

I'm still reading and re-reading this message and not making full sense of it yet; I know there is more to be revealed regarding the energy of separation. To know and feel whole and connected whilst living as a separate being is our journey. I've recently been reading a book by Anna Delves, 'A Memory Returned', about the moment of 'The Split' and mulling over how this fits in with Rosa's messages. The Split moment is when we moved from feeling unity, a whole of light and in balance, into the fragments of light we are now, the illusion of being separate from the whole.

Those who chose to live this separation energy through adoption need to be honoured and supported for their courage and willingness to feel this gaping wound so acutely.

Rosa talks about coming to a place of forgiveness for being separated. I'm a huge fan of forgiveness. It's incredibly powerful to release yourself of the burden of someone else's wrongdoing or perceived wrongdoing – or your own. But telling someone they have to or should forgive doesn't work for me either. I believe we are in a position to forgive when we have worked through the various aspects of the trauma. Forgiving yourself first. Forgiveness is a journey to a place an individual has the potential to reach through finding resolution to the trauma and feeling stronger in ourselves, more whole, not a thing we can just pull out of the blue because someone else thinks it's a good idea. This is how I read Rosa's message: that healing the wounds of separation eventually, at some point, will lead to a time when forgiveness is possible and welcomed and the burden of separation is lifted.

Rosa mentions in her message the need to have a connector and to feel connected. Those who have been adopted can find connection with their adopted parents, but they also need a connection from further back. Adoption is a traumatic event. If we experience trauma, such as a loss, accident or attack, anything that is a threat to life, we have knowledge and awareness of what it felt like to live before that event. Adoptees have no reference point to what life was like before – all they have ever known is the trauma. I feel that if adoptees feel able to move through the painful emotions they experience in this lifetime, they may feel able to connect with their birth mother, energetically at least, through Birth Matrix Reimprinting for one, and if not, travel to past lives where they were loved and find their connection there, or their connection to Source. All is possible when and if the time is right for a person to delve deeply into themselves.

## Back to our why; the role we're playing

Therefore in the bigger, bigger picture, we all have the opportunity to play our part in restoring the earth to its rightful place as the heart of the universe, the planet of love, so it can rise ever higher back to the oneness that is the original energy of creation, the oneness of the energy of the 'big bang'. As we restore ourselves, let go of our old patterns and conditioning, drop the lower energies of betrayal, resentment and guilt, and rise, so does the earth. I feel the earth is rising anyway, with or without us and so our choices in rising with her become more profound.

Where we are heading, or have the potential to head, is to a feeling of oneness whilst living on this planet. Greater unity and cooperation are called for. The masculine energy in us all, and the men here now, must be supported to feel less fearful and therefore less inclined to take and hold onto control. The feminine energy in us all, and all women now, must be supported to feel safe and empowered so they can shine at their brightest. There will be greater balance. The energy of creation will come back into balance. The story of the creation of the universe restored so each of us no longer needs to continually play out the distortion and all that brings.

I am not claiming I've read Rosa's message correctly or interpreted it right. I actually have no need to be right! I'm just putting out the messages that came through me and trying to figure out the story of creation in my small human mind and how it is affecting our daily lives now – a task that I can only play with, and be intrigued by, rather than pinning down truth right now. I'd love to open up discussion so we can all add our knowledge into the pot that will help others understand themselves and their life on a deeper level, to feel lifted, powerful and free to be them – more connected to themselves and ultimately the earth and all the beauty around them. I've added a link at the back of the book to my social media contacts and a Rosa's Choice group where this discussion can continue.

However you read Rosa's message of creation, however you interpret it, is your truth for where you are right now. We are all here to find our own truth when we're ready and not be told what it should mean. It's important to interpret all of Rosa's messages in your own way. The key point throughout this book is to be curious and take responsibility for your own thoughts and feelings, is it your truth or someone else's? This is how you reclaim the fullness and beauty of who you are and step into your power as a creator.

## Who do we blame?

One of the oldest most ingrained beliefs in some religions is that

God, the Creator, punishes and we have to be fearful and reverent and even pay money to avoid these punishments. In times long ago, individuals or churches had the right to intervene in our lives as a middleman between your personal conscious and higher self – as if you weren't worthy, good enough, pure enough, or able to do so in your own right. They had the right to say what was deemed to be good or bad as they saw it – to 'cleanse our souls' into their interpretation of the world otherwise we would not be worthy of God. However, if in fact, we are all and everything, essentially our own Gods co-creating our realities, will we start to take more responsibility for our actions and behaviours?

Is external war merely a reflection of our own inner conflict as we grapple with fear, lack, and powerlessness? The following message, also from Source/Creator/unconditional love/the all and everything – whichever name you put to it – presents us with a different perspective of war. And once again brings us to the truth of who we are underneath all the layers of hatred, bitterness, fear and resentment: we are love and we are joy.

## A message from source on war and joy

Source: Today it is to war and also to joy I would like to turn, and how these two are the same sides of one coin. This may be a difficult concept for you to understand, for where there is war, how can there be joy?

And yet there is. There is joy in the solitary flower that has survived a barrage of gunfire. There is joy in the birth of a child, despite the scenes around them. And there is joy in the hearts of the people who are able to sit in the cafes and along the riversides and meeting places of these venues of war, as they connect for a short time, not with the war, but with themselves and their friends and their families.

Do you see there is always joy, no matter what the experience around you? It is simply a case of noticing it. However, for many of you now, joy seems to be a thing that is not attainable, and is only attainable if attached to money, fame and celebrity, houses, cars, and all the wealth of joy around you, when in fact none of these things are joy; for joy is who you are. It is not something to be bought and treasured and held onto as if your very lives depended on it, but something to be embraced and shared and acknowledged, for joy is everything and as we have said, joy can be found in the most miserable of circumstances.

However, it is more often the case that we don't allow ourselves to feel joy. We don't feel the joy because we don't notice the joy – so busy are we in our minds, searching, always searching, for our fears, the things we believe we don't have, the things we believe we need to have, the things we believe we never had, our perception of loss and lack, that rarely do we see what we do have. And what we do have is joy, because you not only have it, you are it. How is it that you will be able to find your joy, how is that you will be able to find your peace and your joy? Do you know that to do this you only need to find yourself?

There is nothing more to say on this issue. People are joy, joy is people. To find their joy they must find themselves and to find themselves they must go inside and delve beneath the layers of the mind and body and directly into the heart, the heart of the centre of the truth of who you are – at heart.

The more you know of yourself in each moment, the more you will bring joy, bring life, bring love, to the ways of the world that you feel are far from joyful. There is no such situation as joylessness, for where there is life, there is joy.

Even in war, because it makes no matter what situation you are living in or finding yourself in. There is no escaping the fact that you are still joy, no matter what. And often you may not feel this joy. However, that is not to say it is not there. Seek to find your joy in every moment and every moment will therefore be filled with joy.

There will be no joy felt at the loss of a child or a loved one in war, but again, this does not mean that joy is not present. It must be present if you are present. And the life of your child was present. That is joy, for you are nothing but joy, do you see? Even if you cannot possibly feel it, it is there, because it is you.

You are joy, even when, perhaps especially when, it is a feeling that seems out of reach. Even when you are in your darkest depths, that does not mean you are the dark depths. Because you are and always have been and will be, joy.

# Chapter 13
## As Above, So Below.
## Messages from Mother Earth and the galactics

I find myself saying this statement, 'as above, so below', quite often – or the statement that our role here is 'to bring heaven down to earth'. What I mean by this is that your babies are a piece of heaven coming to earth – an energy of pure love – and you, the woman, as the energy of pure love, have the right and ability and power to be the portal and container for this pure love. You are also a piece of heaven on earth.

We always seem to be looking upward or outward to heaven, or wanting to escape somewhere that feels more heavenly, happier, more joyful, really. As the message in Chapter 8 (What does age have to do with it?) states: why would we need to die – to leave here and go somewhere else that seemed less fraught and difficult and dense – if we knew we had the power to create the same feeling here on earth? If the vibration of earth lifted to the high vibration of 'heaven'.

Rosa's message on creation says that there is no above or below. We may look skywards for our answers – to the heavens so to speak – or to our own hearts and wisdom. The message below suggests that our answers can also be found in the earth.

### Connecting with the source of life in earth

We hold both the heavens and the earth in the same consciousness. We can connect with all things and all beings seen or unseen, because we are all things. We have simply been trained out of this knowing.

During a recent meditation in my Divine Mother Meditation Circle, we were taken down and shown the Source energy that resides in the earth, and I saw it exactly the same as I see Source energy when I take my awareness upwards. I experienced this as the great central sun, but in the earth. As above, so below. Rosa is always telling me my answers are in the earth, everything we need to know is in the earth. I'm currently practising, realigning my practise to this. Again, reminding me of turning our beliefs upsidedown.

Anyone with a pet knows the connection they have with animals. Anyone who loves gardening knows their connection with the earth and the plants. It's not seen as weird to love animals and plants, but the moment you mention how you feel and communicate with nature, communicate with the 'other' , feel at one with the 'other', which is not the same as you, not material or physical, the age-old barriers of separation kick in along with fear, shame, humiliation, and lack. We've been trained through fear to see our human selves as different, above and separate, from ourselves, each other, nature, and most certainly with the unseen, the 'other'. We've been trained and humiliated into being disconnected.

The reason, I would argue, is because when people feel more connected to themselves and to others and the world around them, they are far more empowered and therefore far less likely to be told what to do. More easily controlled.

One day, I decided to see what would happen if I connected, really connected, with Mother Earth and the energies and beings of the earth. I did this with no expectation, just simple curiosity about whether it was possible. Sarah Joanne Ashurst, a friend and mentor of each other, has a deep connection to the elemental realms. I'm part of her beautiful elemental Fairy and Angel Academy, where we increase our connection to the realms of the fairies, dragons, sprites and others. One day I simply thought: why not ask the earth for a message and see what happens? Below is what came through.

> It has been for far too long that we have remained hidden from view, hidden from sight, as you chose to see only the plants and the birds and the animals and yet not the very life force that enables these creatures to be. The very life force that indeed creates and allows you to be. So, do you understand how important it is to see, really see, the flowers that are opening up for you and the waves and waters of the world that are the washers of you?

The bees and the insects are the creators and the bin men of the world, because without them, you will not exist, and we are urging you to see this. We are all of the very same life force. And this life force we are holding onto on this planet can and does serve the whole universe.

Do you see how important it is that we are all seen as one? Do you see how vital it is not only that we can see you but that you too are able to see us? See us in the opening of a flower; hear us in the buzzing of a bee. Direct your minds from the fact that we may or may not be here, into a place of simply knowing that we are.

Because we are you and we all thrive on the very same life force that keeps you alive and the very same life force that allows the leaves of the trees to fall away in a gentle cleansing of love only to come back again the next year in full and vital bloom, ever stronger and more vibrant.

All we ask is that you see us. See us in your mirrors and see us in your hearts; see us in your showers in the water that falls down from above, for this very water is blessed whether it is the water of a shower or waterfall out in nature.

So protect these sites and protect yourselves and protect us, for within all of this protection is only love of the highest, most pure vibration. The vibration that is all of life and a life that must and can be sustained through the full acknowledgement of our existence and the existence of all life on earth – a life of joy, a life of wonder, a life of love.

## What have volcanic eruptions got to do with anything?

I went through quite a phase of talking to the earth and I need to continue to practise this connection because the wisdom and messages are extraordinary, messages for the New Earth way of living, because the earth has and is already living that reality. The following message from Source reveals that the wisdom we hold deep in our energetic wombs is the wisdom and secrets of life that have been hiding under the dense layers of energy in the earth. Remember that phrase at the start of this book, that it's through the darkness of the womb we find the light?

In 2018 there was a lot of focus on volcanic eruptions. I'm fascinated by volcanoes anyway but it felt to me like there were an awful lot more eruptions, at least being focused on in the news, at that time. I asked what the deeper meaning of it was. The message from those I call the earth spirits revealed it was all part of a mass awakening, a releasing of layers of energy, and that when these layers were lifted, we'd know the true source of life.

Have a read and, as always, make of it what you will.

## Message from the earth spirits on volcanic eruptions of 2018

Oh, the joy that you recognise we are here with you and that we exist and are here to play and to assist you in your lives, for as you do this, you also assist us. It is with relief and love that we welcome you here today, for it has been a long time in coming, our dearest spirit of the earth.

We have longed for and missed you in our connection and you have been highly resistant to this. But this is of no matter for you were not ready; we were not ready as the world was not ready. And now it is.

It is time to begin the slow road back to self and the slow road back to all that we are, all we have come from – and we are here to show the way. Show the way to lift the layers up from the earth that have kept you stifled, and show you the way up and through these layers you thought were a natural part of human existence, but had in fact been placed there many moons ago, like concrete from your modern times

The earth and the secrets that lie here had to be protected.

Secrets that are now safe to be seen, felt, and revealed. We are in much gratitude of this for it has been many years. Now this concrete can melt and become of the earth itself as we rise up through the layers with our light and information. Our ancient knowledge and worldly ways in order to lead the way to that New Earth that you are all so keen on talking about.

This, my dear, is the New Earth. And, yes, you are one of those who are here to lift the seals that hold you all a step or two away from the real source of the light, the real source of all existence and creativity – for it is a light that resides down here and not up there where you all believe it to be.

So we like to smile at the irony of this and yet you are now all ready to look at this in a very different way. We will do this gently and kindly, for like any old musty secrets, they must first be dusted off, the dust blown away for the true magnificence of it to be revealed, to the fullest of its capacity.

When we were first taken into the light of source itself, the world around us did indeed collapse and tumble into the sea and many mountains formed at this time, adding extra layers of weight and protection to the very sealing of ourselves and the protection of the greatest wisdom that has long been forgotten.

And so it is, we welcome you once again into the fold that is the true humanity of this world and all the secrets of that humanity that can once again be dusted off and revealed to the masses.

I continued to play with connecting with the earth. Whilst on holiday in Croatia, we visited the beautiful and impressive waterfall in Krka National Park. I was mesmerised by the flood of water pouring from the hills and felt alive swimming in the pools at the bottom. Knowing absolutely everything has a purpose beyond what we can physically see and are aware of, the thought crossed my mind to connect in with the earth there and ask what else was going on.

I started to see visions of old conflicts, soldiers and blood being washed away downstream, and was told that the water here, and I assume all water on earth, had a purpose of cleansing away old energies, old traumas and conflicts, washing away negative and stagnant energy.

I'm sure you've all felt how being in water and even near water is reviving – and energetically that's exactly what it does. It supports us not only in the obvious life-giving physical ways, but on a deeper level too.

Doctors are always telling us to drink more water, for obvious reasons. When we feel tired, hungry and unwell, often all we need is more water and a large dose of nature. If water is cleansing the earth of negative energy, when we drink clean water ourselves, we are nourishing our bodies and also helping to remove unwanted and negative energy. Water keeps our energy flowing. It is a vital life source on all levels of our physical and energetic being.

It's worth checking out the work of Dr Masaru Emoto on water if you want to follow up further around this subject.

In one Soul Plan reading, my client and I were shown how she was connected to the River Nile eons ago, directing its waters, energetically being attuned to the water energy, and bringing life to the region. These waters were a sign of the Divine Feminine flowing, the life force energy that sustains abundance along its shores.

I always see water as a feminine energy. We're surrounded in water in the womb and the experience of a water birth by those who have experienced or birthed their own child is one much loved by women and independent midwives. Water has memory, we are drinking and bathing in the same water now as the dinosaurs did, it is recycled. Gifted healer and physic artist Jenny Parris has written a children's book on this topic entitled 'Evo's Travels'. It's a very sweet way of not only understanding the water cycle and how water changes form, but also the journey of life.

It makes me more aware to bless and energetically cleanse the water I drink thinking about all the people, creatures, experiences and lifetimes of energy this water has passed through. Another thought that came to me that I don't have the answer to, but just want to add to the discussion , is that if water is the feminine – our home in the womb is in water and we're birthed into the feminine waters – were water blessings such as baptisms and christenings maybe once another welcome into the feminine energies, to Mother Earth? Up until recently, it used to be only a man who could baptise someone and rather than to the Mother Earth, it was to a patriarchal interpretation of God.

As I've said, it's time to question everything we have been taught, heard and seen as we've grown up. It's time to flip what we think is normal and see it from another perspective, or many perspectives, until we each can find our truth. Flip things a little so that the pendulum swings from upside down to one of balance.

## Turning 'truths' on their head

Sometimes the world appears upside down in how it works. I used to work for an international charity and saw many injustices and upsidedowness on my travels. For example, the local people in places like Africa, countries such as the Congo which is abundant in gold, precious metals and also the coltan needed to run our mobile phones, laptops and tech. Either they risk their lives mining the tiniest amount of these gifts of nature for a pittance, or are paid a pittance from companies. Mother Earth receives nothing for her gifts except poisoned rivers from the cyanide that is used in larger, official company operations to extract the gold.

The earth and those closest to the source of these gifts are at the very tail end of benefitting in all aspects, and anyone who has watched the film 'Blood Diamonds' will be aware of the damage – physical, social, and economic – this upsidedown system creates. How many wars have there been over resources?!

In monetary terms, the benefits to the locals living near the source is a pittance. More goes to the middle-men, more still to the company workers, and then to the shareholders. The ones who are furthest away from the source of these precious metals receive the most. How is that right? Let alone how and why we are poisoning the water sources, the life of the earth because of it. To mine or not to mine is a world issue to address. From my point of view, are there alternatives? If we mine, how can this be done differently? What does a win-win look like for the earth and us all, and not just for the few? I believe the new generations and future generations of children, the New Earth children, if allowed their full, creative expression, will be the ones discovering and implementing new ways.

When looking for a publisher for this book I was astonished at how little the writer receives. One company was paying just 10% of royalties. Amazon took 30 percent and this company the rest. The writer, the source, who relies upon other services to get published, gets taken further and further away from their creation in terms of money. Many musicians, artists, creative people and their endeavours seem to be stuck in this system where they, the creator, the Source, the birther, is not fully acknowledged in this monetary world. The long-held belief of the starving artist is a huge block and it is difficult for many to move out of this mindset. But why is this an image and perception? Is it a truth or is it another reflection for us all to see how the energy of creation is distorted in its value? Thankfully, there are so many different companies flourishing that offer a New Earth way of thinking, a win-win mindset for all. Much like The Unbound Press who published this book.

Is there a different system, a different way of doing things so we as the creators of life we all are, own our own creations and the what, how, if and why we share them?

I've been shown the New Earth Children; your beautiful babies and future babies will be redressing this balance, changing the way business is carried out from competition to cooperation. Introducing new tech that we cannot begin to imagine right now because they won't be stifled by these current systems. Their creative expression needs to be wholly embraced.

The turning things on its head discussion has led me away from where we started on the deeper meaning of water. Who controls access to this life-giving and sustaining element?

Another change of perspective on water which could be helpful is water in the form of rain – especially here in the UK when we can moan about the rain a lot.

On a particularly rainy day, after seemingly weeks and months of rain, I was prompted to ask about the deeper meaning of this type of weather.

**Below is the message from Source.**

> I would like to share with you about the rain. Because all I hear from you is, the rain is this and the rain is that, but have you ever stopped to wonder about the rain? What is the rain? Where does it come from and why is it here?
>
> Do you know that every droplet of rain contains an essence of yourself? An essence of the spirit of life that keeps your earth turning? And in so doing is nourishing to plants, trees and animals, yes, but also to your human lives. Is it not washing away the sadness that a raindrop can bring? Is it not rinsing and cleansing the earth of the darker power of energies that like to keep you separate from the earth and separate from the very life on earth around you?
>
> Imagine not a single droplet of rain fell on you in all of your lifetime. What would you be missing in your life? You'd be missing a cleansing, a purifying, a freedom of standing out in life as you, the very essence of a life pouring along your body, washing the grit from your eyes and the debris from your body.
>
> Yes, this rain is good for your earth, but, my dears, it is also time to know that it is indeed very good for all of you humans too, for without it, there is a harshness to life, a bareness to the life you see before you and a certain sense of hopelessness.
>
> So, do not distract yourselves from the rain and do not 'diss' the rain, for remember the rain is more than just a cloudburst. It is more than a drenching and a soaking and an inconvenience. The rain is a clearing, a cleansing, a force

to bring forth life, bring forth new life, not only in the ground and the soil but also within your soul.

Know the rain is also you and the life you bring, and know also that the rain is bringing you to a new life as the seeds of evil that were planted on your planet many, many moons ago are consistently and lovingly being washed away by the very drops of life force that they bring with them.

So, please welcome the rain and please welcome the clearing for it is only then that the loving sun can truly rise in tandem with it as opposites of the same life-giving force.

It is to welcome all of your experiences in life, as in all weathers there is all beauty and all of life. You are a part of this life and so too must be welcomed in all of your guises and experiences in order for the axis of the world to keep turning, in a way that is very much in favour of life, and very much in favour of you, our dearest souls.

And so it is with love and gratitude I send this message. For all of the wet days that are clearing the way for a much brighter dawn, and an altogether much brighter future.

And so it is.

## Messages from Mother Earth

Once tuned in, the messages from the earth are all around you. It's simply like learning a different language. Those moments of stillness you feel in nature, this is connection. The colour and smell of a flower and how it makes you feel, this is connection. It's not hard. It's about giving yourself a few moments of time to notice, without 'trying' – just being.

Whenever I'm feeling overwhelmed, I always turn to nature and to trees in particular. I have a few favourite trees near to where I live. I have a favourite oak tree and everyone I know in the area also seems to know and is drawn to this tree. Whether or not they are as 'weird' as I am and talk to it, or believe in the healing powers of trees, they don't question why they're drawn to it – they instinctively know it makes them feel better. This magnificent tree has the most incredible energy and I see it as a Divine Masculine tree.

This is a huge oak tree with so many heavy branches reaching out and up. One day when I was feeling particularly stressed and overwhelmed with everything I felt I had to do, I had to get out and go for a walk. I asked this tree what was it I needed to know. The reply: "You may have many branches and can be pulled in many different directions, but you can always stay strong and rooted at your core."

Another tree, interestingly on the other side of my local common, almost directly opposite the oak tree, is one I refer to as the Divine Mother tree. When I lean into her branches I receive image after image of Divine Mother wisdom. It sounds totally bonkers, I know, but this tree gives me messages and I always connect in with her before I lead one of my Divine Mother meditations so I have an inkling of where the healing may be coming from that evening. The book by Peter Wohlleben, 'The Hidden Life of Trees,' scientifically explores the ways in which trees cooperate and network with each other. The message one day from the Divine Mother tree was: "We are not only the guardians of the earth; we are the guardians of you." The subsequent group meditation where we were connected into the tree network was beyond powerful. Sharon McErlane, who is known across the world for her channelling of 'the Grandmothers' and creating a network of light, shared this message about the trees:

> The life force in the trees will harmonise with your own life force. Tune into us at all times. When this happens, you will see things differently, understand in a different way. Let the trees teach you.

This is what is happening for me and many others and it still blows me away. I still question if what I'm hearing or seeing is actually happening, but the point is, it's possible. We are all connected energetically. You can tune into myriads of radio stations through various energetic frequencies; you can't see them, you turn a dial and you're in. In London, you have access to loads of radio stations but as you go further from the centre you can only pick up the nearest local radio station. It's the same when tuning into any frequency. This is how I see channelling: it's tuning into a frequency and translating the energy into one you understand. When I connect in with Rosa's energy, I see it as turning the dial high enough to listen to a local radio station in New Zealand, for example. We all have this ability because we are connected to everything; we're of the same consciousness.

Wherever you're at with your connection, it's all about playing, being curious, because why not? You have absolutely nothing to lose by playing, and so much to gain.

## Message from Source – walking with the earth

You are not walking on the earth, you are walking with the earth, as the earth begins to reclaim its stance and its stand as the heart of the entire universe.

Do not think it is only you humans who have a right to be on this earth and do not think it is only you humans who have a chance at making or breaking this earth. There are very many creatures and very many beings for whom the healing of the earth and the knowing of the earth for what it truly is, is a key they wish to unlock.

Our question to you is: would you rather be working in tandem with all of the creatures for whom the earth is king or queen? Or would you rather continue to work alone, strive alone and battle alone, fighting each other for the land, space, greed and the un-joy of walking on this planet?

Or would you choose, if you could, to walk with joy and not on the earth but with the earth as it rises into the full glory from whence it came? And how does this feel, my dear ones – to rise with the earth as it rises and to see how far and how high you can go with this earth?

Or is it that you choose us to remain here? Simply on the earth with no place other to go than down into its centres, only to be brought back up another time to try again to see that the earth is far more than you think it is, is far more than you know it to be?

It is time to know it. We ask you to look deeply and closely at your lives, and the life around you, and see where it is rising and see where it is falling and make another choice. The choice to choose, the choice to know, and the choice to rise alongside and with the earth and not in a battle over it or upon it.

For as you rise, so does the world. And as the world rises, so do you. For you are one. And there is no other way.

With all of our love. Your guardian spirits and angels upon high and low.

And so it is.

## Hippie, eco warrior, or simply connected?

It is becoming trendy and more acceptable now to be concerned with the environment and nature. Being a tree hugger and someone who loved nature was once dismissed as being a hippie, a weirdo. People were branded and ridiculed for their connection with nature and therefore the sense of separation grew. No one wants to be humiliated and shamed and ostracised for not running with the rest of the disconnected pack.

Now there is a pride in being an eco-warrior, someone who cares about Mother Earth, her seas and her atmosphere – our source of life. What a huge crazy messed-up mind-trick to stop us seeing and feeling our connection to our very source of life, and all because of fear and imbalance of power. A twisted need to dismiss the female, control the 'mother', Mother Earth as the feminine aspect of creation.

It is the young people who are leading the way in this change of perception from weirdo to warrior. And it is your children and future children who will continue bridging this gap between human and nature, bridging the gap between heaven and earth to create heaven on earth, meaning a place of love which is less dense and therefore less difficult to live on. A place of connection.

Have you wondered why there's a surge in unicorn, dragon, and mermaid toys and themes – they're everywhere! I believe this energy is no longer hidden – the realm of the elementals is opening up for us all to recognise, as you'll read a little further on. Real or imagined, the images of these beings bring the energy of joy, playfulness, protection and magic, certainly to our children. And that is the point: they remind us of who we are.

Below is the message that came through from the beings I refer to as the earth spirits. All they are asking is for you to notice the earth, notice the world for all it is and all it provides. Not only does this help the earth to heal, but also us.

We welcome you, our child of light, all our children of light, to this planet you call Earth. It is good to connect in with you again for you have ignored us for quite some time now. You seem to be more aware of us too – and this is a good thing – for we are becoming more and more visible – not only to you, but to all of you.

Have you noticed maybe that the grass looks greener? The sky bluer? The flowers and the plants, the trees and the hedgerows more vibrant than ever before? That the birdsong seems sweeter and the meow of a cat louder, more piercing? If you have not, maybe you should look now. Maybe it is time to notice all the signs and the stars as well as the earth.

All the answers to the universe are here, right here, if only you cared to look and to notice. Yet you are all so busy with your phones and your computers and taking life out of the earth that you do not notice the life that is the earth.

The life that is your earth, the life and the life force that you lie upon, rely upon. The earth on which you build your own life as we support you in our total joy to come and live the lives you wish to live. But we cannot hold this love for much longer without it being replenished.

By this, all we mean is by being noticed. For we ask nothing more than to be noticed. Notice the creatures, notice the plants, notice the noises and the smells and the heartbeat of the earth, the heartbeat of nature and all it is, because when you notice, we notice.

We notice that this is with love and therefore the love we give is more fully recycled into the absolute abundance that is the mother of all mothers, the heart of your planet and the heart of you. We are in honour of you and of your knowing that you are already the abundance that you seek, because you are indeed part of the all and everything of the all and everything.

It is simple: we love you, you love earth and all that is, and life and the life force that this is continues to play and deliver in the abundance that you deserve.

Such a beautiful message, eye-opening and inviting you to take a moment to see, really see, the beauty of the earth. To notice how lying out in the sun on a beach and hearing the waves lapping against the shore makes you feel, or walking in nature. There's a reason why doctors of all specialisms are now recommending more time in nature for emotional and physical well-being. It helps you to feel connected. Unlike walking through a busy shopping centre where we're picking up all sorts of energy from other people, which can lead us to becoming stressed and not knowing why, when we're out in nature we are receiving only good vibes. It's safe to expand our energy wider when we're out in nature.

## Rosa on nature

Today I would like to share with you about nature, about all the world that is around you each and every day and yet often you do not stop to see it or sense it and certainly not often to love it or live it.

For, yes, we do live this nature and although many of you choose to see yourselves as above nature and even beyond the laws of nature, I assure you that you are not, for you are only the size of an insect that is easily squashed as you so often do yourselves to the creatures you call insects.

And does this sound like a harsh thing to you? A wrong thing to say? For if it does then you too surely have this arrogance in you that is currently being healed across the world. This arrogance that deems you to be bigger and better and brighter and lighter than anything else on your planet.

And yet you are not. For you could no more live without the bees and the trees than the very air you breathe. And so do you see why it is so important to look up and look out and look in for all of it is a part of life and none of it can be brought or bought, it merely is.

And that includes you, my dearest of humans, for even though you often don't see yourselves as a part of nature, this is what you are. A part, not apart.

For you are life and they are life and it is life and all is life and you are no greater or smaller than the smallest of creatures you see under your microscopes. Do you not see you are under the microscope too? The microscope of yourself as a Soul who wishes to do much in this world, move gently through this world learning your lessons and sharing your joys and becoming intimate with your sorrow.

For this too is life and this too is nature and the ups and the downs and the ins and the outs, the living and the dying and the growth and re-growth and all that the Universe does, you too experience.

And it is time to see yourselves as such. Not separate, as above or below, but as a part of the very breathing in and breathing out of the Universe itself. And wouldn't life feel so much easier and so much in joy and enjoy-full if you found yourself able to flow in and out with the very tides of the Universe itself?

For this is who you are.

Close your minds and open your hearts, never be afraid to hear the sounds of nature that surround you, for you are the very breath of air that they breathe and they are the very breath of air that you breathe.

So sit still in the waters of your soul and allow the sounds of nature to fill you. To fill in the depth of the hole that sees you feeling separate from nature and separate from the world. Because the truth is, you are far from separate from it, you are it.

Close your minds and open your hearts and listen to your heart as you listen to the sounds of nature. Get to know your unique beat and rhythm. For that is what you are: a sound, a wave, a movement of energy adding your own sound and breath of life to the sounds and breath of the universe and the orchestra that is life itself.

## What is grounding and why is it important?

If there is one thing for you to do every day in terms of self-care, grounding is the one I would go to. Grounding is when, with intention, you feel yourself connecting with the earth, sending your energy down through the soil. Children instinctively know this and love to run about barefoot on the grass or soil or sand.

There have been a few scientific studies on grounding and tests run on patients with, for example, cardiovascular disease, to discover the benefits for health. Grounding, or earthing, helps your own electrical impulses to become more balanced, equalised with the earth's electrical potential. In other words, it calms down your nervous system through a transfer of electrons from the earth to the body.

A study on the website healthline.com/health/grounding, measured blood measurements taken before and after grounding to determine any changes in red-blood-cell fluidity, which plays a role in heart health. The results indicated significantly less red-blood-cell clumping after grounding, which suggests benefits for cardiovascular health. Grounding is a great way to de-stress. Yay to the science that shows us what we already innately know. Children love running about barefoot and they also love being in water. It's time to look more deeply at what our children are teaching us about our connection to the earth. And the new souls arriving will be even more in need and in knowing of their connection to nature.

## Heart to heart with baby

Whilst talking about your electrical impulses, it seems a good time to bring us back a moment to women and babies – to whom this book is dedicated. There is also so much science now about the electrical impulses of our hearts and how important a heart-to-heart connection between mum and baby is for life. This is why placing baby in mum's arms skin-to-skin and heart-to-heart following birth allows for all sorts of magical physiological responses to occur for the health and well-being of mum and baby. Sleeping in the same room as your baby helps hearts keep beating and connecting.

Someone I know who works with children experiencing developmental delays shared a story of one child who was pronounced dead soon after his arrival. He is now fully flying without any extra support and is up to speed with what is considered 'normal' in terms of development phases. His distraught mum instinctively asked to hold him and when the doctors lifted his little body off the resuscitation table and placed him in his mum's arms, after a short while, his heart began beating. Scientifically and energetically this is possible as the electrical impulses from her heart fired up the electrical impulses in his heart. Truly the miracle of life and connection we have with our children. We are One.

## Universal support and connection

So you now know that you support you. You are your own universe and the Universe. You support others. Source energy supports you. And the earth supports you. You support and support others and are supported in all ways by all things seen and unseen because you are connected and a whole part of an even bigger whole. You are made of the same source, the same energy.

To really push the boat out now, the earth and therefore we, are also affected and supported by many other beings. It's common knowledge how the phases of the moon affect the seas and our emotions. The earth is a part of a bigger whole, other planets, other universes. As we're all connected and have an effect on each other, when the earth is in trouble, that likely means they are feeling the effects. So why wouldn't they want to play a part in the rebalancing and rising of the earth? There are many lightworkers spreading messages from what are collectively called the galactics. The Pleiadians, Sirians, Lyrans, and Arcturians to name a few. There is a huge amount of literature out there. Right now I'm intrigued about learning more about this bigger picture and what it offers us and I'm testing the water to find my own truth in it. All I can speak about is from my own personal experience.

One moment that comes straight to mind, and still blows my mind, is connecting in with a spirit baby who had chosen not to stay – her energy was unlike anything I'd felt before and I was told this was the energy of a highly evolved soul – Arcturian energy. Both myself and her mum felt the sheer power of love emanating from her, which is impossible to describe. Another moment was in my Divine Mother Meditation circle when a being saying they were from the Pleiades popped in to offer some healing. Again, an extraordinary energy that was felt by each member of the group.

I've channelled messages from these energies, met people who hold this energy, and travelled with clients to other planets to explore their lives there and why this is relevant for them to know at this point in time. It is truly a beautiful, loving energy. But just as there is light and dark here on earth, I'm assuming the same goes for 'out there'. Always be discerning as to who you are sharing your energy with, whether human or un-seen energies. I have my own ritual of always connecting in with Source first to ensure only the highest connection serving love. Really, love is your greatest protection, there is no greater force in the universe than the intention of coming from love for the highest and best good of all.

Below is a message via Source on the support offered by our galactic friends. And perhaps another piece in the puzzle as to why the earth became a place of such imbalance, as was mentioned in Rosa's message on creation when she spoke about those newcomers to earth who didn't understand how it operated. Make of it what you will! I just thought it was a good place to begin closing up this bigger, bigger and ever more bigger picture of the universe.

**Alien support message from those who call themselves the masters and co-creators of the Universe**

Our gods and goddesses of earth, we are here to honour you and assist you in the rising and the reclamation of your planet as the heart and truth of the universe. A planet that has long been shadowed by the plague of darkness that we ourselves once brought to you from our other realms.

But we are here now. And we are with you now in love and gratitude, our beings of light, in honoured service to the world within worlds in which we operate. We offer our utmost sadness and ask for forgiveness up to the realms of the Almighty God of all Gods for all that has come to pass in our experimentations of life and love that have so fully added to the darkness of the world.

As we forgive ourselves and are forgiven, it is in the rising and redemption, the love and the truth of the light that exists within you all that will be upheld and uploaded from the very caverns of the earth and back into the light and love of the earth itself.

It is our utmost wish and desire to be here to serve you now in this way in the turning of the world from the darkness and back into the light where it once was. To restore order and fairness, the balance between the light and the dark of which there cannot be one without the other.

The light that we now honour and uphold, not the dark, for you have shown us the way with your faith and your duty and your honour and your love for the earth and each other and the selves that you are.

We come now to help you restore and to be restored into the fullness of who you are, a fullness that was once taken from you and a fullness that was once hidden from you in order to meet our own ends.

However, we realise that our own ends will never be met, for there is no end, there are only constant beginnings. And we are asking to join you now in your New Beginnings from a place of love and gratitude; a place of depth and true learning of what it means to be a part of this great and miraculous universe that is here for all of us to give and receive, and not to be taken from and controlled.

This is no more. We are bored with the battle now of the light and the dark and we have a sense of ennui about what we have been and are about. And we choose now to join you instead in the light. We return to you everything that we have taken and everything that we took from a place of darkness and evil and power and greed and the resentment and the envy that lay within us.

And we only did so in order for you too to feel both the joys and the horrors of these emotions. And yet now this no longer needs to be the way that we operate or that life operates. For as we have learnt, so have you. As we have become bored of the patterns and the constant pretence, so have you.

It is time now for a truce and for us all to surrender. To surrender to the pure joy of what is. And we can welcome you into our world now without fear of the darkness – for the darkness was for us, the light.

We are asking you now to welcome us into your world without fear.


## Universal Oneness – is it possible?

In truth, we are all one. In truth, we are all of the light and the dark and there is no other way to be, other than to be in this truth and at peace with this truth. Then there will surely be no more need for the battle. Neither the battle within nor the battle without.

For there will be harmony as the worlds of light and dark come together in all the colours of the rainbow. A rainbow of colour so bright that there will never again be a dark day of fighting, for there is no longer anything to fight for. The battle is won and there are no losers, for there is no such thing.

For in this world, there are only the learners and the learnt, the masters and the students, who will continue to rise as one into the truth of all truths. The truth that is God and the universe. The truth of the all and everything of the all and everything.

As students of this truth, we are to become the masters of it. And that is our mission. And that is our joy. And we bless you with the unveiling of this truth in the most practical and loving of ways imaginable.

As we are you.

And so it is.


It may also seem odd to end this book with a message that mentions the word evil! It's an awful word that conjures up all sorts of fearful images for me. But if we remember what Rosa's words and the messages from Source and other light beings have been offering, it's a different perspective. A way of looking at the world that draws attention to the false beliefs we may be carrying about ourselves and the way the world works. The messages cut through these beliefs to help you be curious about what feels right for you and not what we've carried through from others. The messages are intended to help you see yourself more clearly.

I hope the following message from Source will turn around the story of evil from one that is something you have no power over and have to battle against, to one of possibility and that you have a choice in. Evil and veil are made up of the same letters.

## Lifting the veils of illusion

Evil is not a thing, nor an act, it is more of a veil, a veil of illusion that keeps you from seeing the full truth, the whole truth. It is this veil that has led to many things happening in your world that can be condemned as 'evil' – an evil – a veil – that shows only the harshness of this side of life and not the beauty that is the truth of all of life.

Do you see that when this veil is removed, as is being so at this time, you will all be able to see that the world can live without this evil, this veil of illusion that keeps you from knowing the whole truth of who you are at heart, our dearest of Souls on this extraordinary planet of earth.

You will once again see life beyond the veil as it is washed and cleansed by the love that is being felt and experienced across the planet by a whole host of beings for whom we are forever grateful.

You are one of these beings of love who has a choice in lifting off your own veils of illusion to see the truth of who you are. A challenging journey to motherhood is one of the opportunities you have to clear the smudges off the window that life has left there, so you have a clearer view. Your babies are helping to remind you of your truth and your role as they prepare themselves to play their part in building a New Earth. A world of unity, love, and connection.

# Chapter 14
# Conclusion

I'm not really sure how to follow that last message, or how to finish this book. I still find it quite mind-blowing when I think back to my heartbroken self who only wanted to become a mum without all the fear, pain and loss, without the bitterness and the shame and every other emotion it brought up in me. How all of those experiences have led me to writing this book.

I'm writing this final chapter from a hotel room on my home island of Jersey, exactly nine years to the day that I released Rosa. The timing of its completion is not lost on me! Nine is also the number of completion. I'm over here to celebrate a friend's birthday, but I know there's a deeper meaning to me being here at this time.

Arriving yesterday, I had to take a look again at the deep sense of loss, love and gratitude for my gorgeous grandparents and my incredible mum and dad. My life here growing up on the beaches, and the freedom I had. The person I thought I was, growing ever more into the person I am. Being in my childhood place with old friends knowing I am still the same, but so different. Letting go of the me I thought I was. I feel Rosa and my loved ones here with me in the room as I write my final words, tears streaming down my face, carrying a tinge of sadness, a little terror, but mostly relief, awe, gratitude and excitement. They are willing me to finish, willing me to be me. As I am inviting you to do the same – be you.

I'm also still not quite sure how it's all happened that my original idea for the book to help ease some of the pain and create a deeper understanding for women on challenging journeys to motherhood has developed into a book about creation itself!

I have gone through an inner conflict at bringing Rosa's messages to light, and it's been another challenging journey birthing this creation. I have no idea who will read it, or where it will go. No idea of how people will receive the messages, whether readers will be welcoming, hostile or indifferent. And the really great thing is that I have no expectations. I feel my job is to share the messages, show up and physically write and create and publish this book. The rest is up to Rosa, the new souls arriving, and how the energy flows in the universe.

I have translated Rosa's messages and those of the other beings who showed up to be a part of this book and share their insights. I'm bringing my own knowledge and experiences to the book that must inevitably be very different from yours. How I've interpreted the messages may not be how you would interpret them. We'll all read them differently depending on our own life experiences and how we see the world. But my wish is that, at the very least, you are curious about what they might mean for you, how they make you feel, and that you might find your own truth within them.

And for those of you who are here to support the women of light and the souls here to build a New Earth, I hope this book will help you to recognise the beauty and magnitude of your work.

Spirits often say to me, we can't do this alone. We need you, people in physical form, to work with us. They need us to take action. We all have a very important role to play, whether you are aware of it or not. I know that maybe right now your own individual pain in regard to becoming a mum may not be eased by the great work you have chosen to do on a soul level. But please know you are not only becoming a mum, you are becoming you.

Your challenging journey to motherhood is pushing you to dig deep inside yourself, to truly know yourself and break free of this lifetime's, and ancient lifetimes', patterns of being powerless, being less than, not knowing you are a creator. The challenge of your journey is gifting you with the opportunity to know yourself on a deeply profound level as a person and as a portal so loving, so courageous, so powerful that you are able to invite, hold, and transform energy into form, and to birth new life, new consciousness, into the world.

You need you. Your babies need you. And the earth needs you to know just how incredible, magical and miraculous you are. You don't need to get your head around all the messages in this book until you want to or need to. You don't need to do anything other than allow yourself the opportunity to unravel all that life has shown you and find the truth of you within it. There'll be a right time for you to open up to the bigger mysteries of the universe. For now, all you need to know is: it all starts with you.

Earlier, when I needed to stretch my legs and take in a bit of sea air, I 'happened' to go into a café I'd never been in before for a coffee and I 'happened' to sit at the only table with a copy of the local newspaper, the Jersey Evening Post, which I used to write for myself. The opinion page was written by Dr Patricia Tumelty, a systemic psychotherapist, and a statement halfway through her article jumped out at me. She was quoting influential educator Paulo Freire: "The dream of a better world runs the risk of idealising a better world or becoming submerged in fatalism, both of which are alienating positions. It follows that accepting the dream that things will come together for the better, requires accepting the process of its creating."

Your babies and future babies, and – whether you know it or wish to know it or not – you, are here to change the world and build a New Earth. They are highly evolved souls coming in with a very high vibration. They are connected to Source and likely many will remember their connection and their missions – unlike ourselves who experienced the amnesia that comes when we arrive and spend our lives trying to remember who we are. In order to do that, you, all of us, have to find ways to accept where we're at now, individually and as a collective, and where the world is at.

It has taken us thousands of years to get to where we are now from the moment people put a border around a piece of land and laid claim to it and later in time began to exploit it. Climate change is a well-worn phrase and one that is also separating. What does it actually mean to the average person on the street? We are talking about the air we breathe that allows life to continue, the seas and waters that cleanse and provide, the earth that is giving and abundant. Biodiversity and wildness are being lost at an alarming rate whilst politicians focus on the economic. Patriarchy is being shown up for what it truly is – disconnected and controlling and based on fear of lack. It is a way of being, an energy that is well past its sell-by date.

I believe it is time for us to wake up. Time to re-examine our own beliefs, habits and learning and replace them with kinder more harmonious thoughts and practices. It's time for us to take responsibility for how we feel and react, find our connection with ourselves, which in turn will reconnect us with the feminine, rebalance the masculine within us, and reconnect us with the mother of all mothers, Mother Earth.

We are entering the time of the rise of the Mother God, the mother god that is you, the mother god that is the earth.

My heartfelt wish is that through the pain you come to joy, that you hold your babies in your arms, or meet them in spirit and understand why they chose not to stay.

With all our love and blessings on your journey,

Debra and Rosa.

# Your multidimensional self – stepping into a new way of being

## An additional message from Rosa on - The Present Moment

So I am here to tell you about the present, there is no such thing for you are here and everywhere all at the same time.

There is nothing that is going on that is not happening in other places and other times and in other lives than right now. The present you are experiencing is just a glimpse of this moment in time in your consciousness as you see it right now. Other parts of you are experiencing many different lives and experiencing this same moment but in very different ways. And that is why we cannot hold onto the present for it is happening many times over as we live different lives and make the many different choices we have at our disposal.

This concept of time is irrelevant here where I sit, for I can see all moments in time. This is why your concept of the present moment is now defunct and past 'its time'. We are living a multitude of lives in a multitude of moments in a multitude of worlds and each is bringing something to your soul. Imagine if your soul could connect all of these moments into one big explosion of knowingness, of concept, of understanding of who you truly are? Your mind would likely explode as this is far too huge and far too much 'energy' for you to be able to contemplate in your earth plane.

And so it is that your present moment is merely a snapshot of what is really going on in the world. If we could all align our present moments from across lifetimes then this is what you would call God. The energy of all-knowing and all-seeing and all possibility.

How would that sit with you? How would that change how you live your life? How would that change how you treat others? Are they merely just the ones who haven't been able to draw back their present moments into one, amalgamous, all-seeing, all-knowing creature that need not worry about anything, or feel the need to experience everything and have everything because they already know they have it all and are experiencing it all at the same time?

If you could imagine being and having and knowing everything, would have little to strive for on earth and so would wish to return home. And so your soul is separated into tiny pieces, each piece living in their own moment, in order to bring that experience back to the whole, where they will one day merge together and therefore all will be done and our work and your work will be done and we will be together again once more.

Do you understand that what I am saying here is that each and every one of you is part of the same whole, the same Soul, that splits off to experience their one moment of insanity or bliss with the one purpose of bringing that back to the core and becoming whole once more.

So you am I, and I am you, and your neighbour is part of You, as is your friend and so too is your enemy. They are all one and the same and so how sad and ironic it is that you choose to end the moments of some souls before they have a chance to complete their piece in the puzzle, which would have helped you to become whole, no matter whether you thought what they were doing in that moment was right or wrong.

And so it is that your present moment is important, but so is the present moment of all your souls, and how you interact with them can either help or hinder your own mission. You are not only your present moment, but you are also theirs. And so through theirs, you will grow, and through yours, so will they.

It is time now to grow together and help each other in our present moments of joy or bliss or death and sadness as they are not just theirs but yours. If your mission is to become whole, then help others to become whole by also 'being' their present moment for them and with them, for they are you and you are them.

Small snippets of the whole bringing back information and knowledge and experience to the greater being that is God.

It is not only your present moment that is important but everybody else's too. If this was the case would you not ensure that everyone is living in a state of present moment bliss so this is what you too feel?

The more of you that live with this wider knowledge connection of who you are and what you are aiming to achieve, the greater the bliss of the whole. By helping each other live more at ease in their present moments, then the more at ease you too shall feel.

## I asked - Who is this message for?

This message is for anyone who cares to listen to it and understand it. There are many so-called 'light workers' on your planet and they are looking for new ways to reach out and do this. The more this message is spread – helping yourself, helps others, helps you – a new wave of understanding will come as to why they are doing what they are doing. They are ultimately helping themselves to become whole because we are all indeed one.

## I asked - Is this Ho' openhopono?

Ho'openhopono is one way of doing this, yes, and the closest one to what I am saying here, but it must now go a step further. It must be brought to the masses as an everyday occurrence that people see themselves in everyone around them and do their best to ensure that others are enjoying their present moment, feel good in their bodies and in their lives as they are merely part of your own experience, and if you choose to experience life in a certain way, in a higher way, then you must help others to do the same because their present moment is also yours.

And so the present moment does not exist as you see it now in your breathing and living, for it means nothing without the presence of others' present moments being the same. Change your perception of others and you change your perception of yourself, for they are merely just another part of you.

I am present in each and every one of your present moments, for I, too, am you.

# I asked - how does this relate to our book about baby souls?

This is all about baby souls because baby souls are merely part of you wishing to come down to join you in this game of wholeness and to add their own unique mix into the mix, and be part of this huge experience of energies and all experiencing the same, which is ultimately nothing but love and joy.

The baby souls are seeking love and joy and to be part of that, and this new wave of souls all they want to do is offer light so all people can experience the oneness from which they come.

In terms of your book, I am a mere guide, and perhaps not what you thought I would be or would be offering. But you have a big task to fulfil and that is to let humanity know that the light is coming and it is coming in waves of love to lift them out of this current mode of selfishness and your concept of oneness – as in 'I am the One' – to a concept of Oneness that is 'We are the One'.

Our journey together sowed the seeds for this and so it is. Go with it, go with me with trust that it is time to reveal the secrets of the Universe at a higher level than the earth has ever known before except in a handful of souls who have been leading the way and treading this path over centuries and generations.

You are a channel and we are love and so together our journey will set the pace for a new way of being. Share what you like but don't jump too soon and lose the momentum of these words, they are designed to run a particular course and you will be guided as to the how and the when.

# I asked - How can I explain this is to do with your choice?

It was my choice to seek a channel for my words and who better than you, my loyal and trusted soul guardian, mate, sister, brother, lover, and lifelong friend. And so it was my choice to come to you and it was your choice to accept me and this is a contract and a love that was formed many eons ago. I would not be talking to you right now if I had not come to you the way I did. And you would not be talking with me now if I had not come to you the way I did.

# Biography

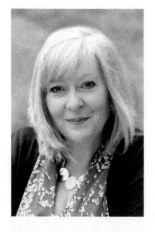

Debra Kilby is a spirit baby medium, conscious conception specialist, channel, healer and spiritual guide. Debra supports women on their journey to motherhood, whether they are struggling to conceive, have experienced baby loss or a traumatic birth. Debra's own challenging journey to motherhood through birth trauma, three miscarriages, and a medical termination, catapulted her into her spiritual awakening and discovering her life purpose. Her Soul's contract is to bring women, their babies and future babies together. To heal the deep wounds of the Mother and the Divine Feminine within this lifetime and others and reawaken the knowledge and wisdom of the New Earth within the wombs of all women. Through deep, loving inner exploration, Debra guides women to transform their perception and understanding of themselves and their journey, and helps them to move from a place of questioning and pain to one of freedom, self-awareness, belief and empowerment. To knowing themselves as loving and powerful creators of life with the ability to hold and birth the energy of new life. Debra works alongside spirit babies to help their mums see themselves as they see them – love.

# Exercises and meditation links to practice to help you with healing and connection

**Meditation to meet your spirit baby for loss and conception**
**https://bit.ly/38hVLsJ**

**Exercise 1**

Give yourself permission to take 20 minutes or so just for you. Create a space, just for you. That might include lighting a candle and creating an altar or it might not – wherever you are, YOU are. Wherever you are, your babies are.

Take three deep breaths imagining you're breathing in the light and this light is moving all the way around your head, down your spine to your feet, and back up to breathe out.

On the third breath let out a deep sigh and allow the weight of your mind to slip down into your chest, your heart chakra.

From your heart, command your energy to zero point. Then command your energy to ground, and finally command your energy to Source.

Set the intention of connecting in with pure unconditional love of Source and imagine yourself sitting under a waterfall of light, cleaning and cleansing your energy and surrounding you in love.

You can ask to connect in with your spirit baby or your higher self or any light being for guidance on any question you may have, or just allow whatever it is that wants to flow through you to flow down the crown of your head, your arm, your hand and onto the page. Start writing, even if it feels like gobbledygook at first, it's a practice.

## Exercise 2

Our beliefs and experiences about what it means to be a mother can affect us in becoming mothers. Write down the word 'mother' on a piece of paper and notice how you feel. Begin writing all the adjectives that come to mind, positive and negative, on what this means to you.

## Exercise 3

Take a moment to feel into this energy of the Divine Mother – unconditional love. Feel held, safe and loved. Call on the energy of the Divine Mother to surround you now.

## Exercise 4

Take a moment to feel into where you are giving yourself a hard time, telling yourself you can't or you're rubbish or limiting yourself.

1. Write in one column all the negative thoughts about yourself. Say them over and over again until you feel bored of them.

2. Ask yourself if this thought is true.

3. In another column, write down a more positive thought.

## Exercise 5

Take some time to write down your journey to motherhood so far, how you feel, what you think about yourself, what you're making it mean about you.

Reflect on how it's changed your life in both positive and negative ways. Notice what you'd like to focus on and change and how you'd like to feel instead.

**Exercise 6**

Notice which thoughts and emotions keep coming back to you. Be curious about these emotions, when's another time you felt them. Who do you blame? Who are you angry at? Or are you blaming yourself? Are you playing the martyr or the victim?

We all have these stories playing out in our minds and they are so very far from the truth of you, the light of you. And those stories can change as you recognise and accept the hugely powerful soul that you are.

**Exercise 7**

It's also beautiful to write a letter to your baby in spirit, pouring out your heart to them. You can then burn this letter and allow the energy to drift up into the realms either for releasing or with the intention of it reaching your spirit baby. Or you can plant it in the soil beneath a beautiful flower or tree and ask the earth to help you connect.

**Exercise 8**

Something you can play with when you feel low or confused is to light a candle and stare into the flame. Allow the light to help fizzle away any negative emotions. You can also ask to be shown visions in the flame too. And if you don't have a candle, your imagination is everything. Close your eyes and imagine gazing into the flame, it's the same effect.

**Exercise 9**

To practise 'hearing' your spirit baby, give yourself some space, light a candle, and imagine you're sitting in a noisy coffee shop. Invite them to join you and imagine you have to lean over the coffee table and focus all your attention on hearing them. Within that silence, you can hear the voice of your spirit baby.

## Exercise 10

Notice the signs and ask for signs from your spirit baby, they are all around you. If there's a bird or animal, a flower or cloud, a rainbow, a number, or song on the radio that grabs your attention, there are infinite ways your baby is communicating with you. You'll know it's a sign from them because of how they make you feel.

## Stay in touch with me

**www.debrakilby.com**

Facebook: Debra Kilby Healing

Instagram: debrakilbyhealing

LinkedIn: Debra Kilby

**To join in more discussion on Rosa's Choice, request to join here: https://bit.ly/2WwAMNm**

## Work with me

**Courses:**

Sacred Conception: A New Dawn. Birthing the Children of the New Earth:

https://debrakilby.com/sacred-conception/

From Here to Maternity. 7 Steps to Meeting Your Baby: Healing Mind, Body and Soul for Conception:

https://debrakilby.com/2020/04/01/from-here-to-maternity/

A New Dawn. Birthing Women of the New Earth. A journey back to truth, love and the ancient wisdom of self.

Take a look at my website debrakilby.com for more information.

**Work with me One to One**

www.debrakilby.com or email me at: Debrakilbyhealing@gmail.com

Join myself and other women in our Divine Mother Wisdom membership group.

A space for women to gather, share and receive love, wisdom and gifts with a monthly circle as well as healing meditations and channelled messages from the Divine Mothers.

Please message me or go to my website for more information. Debrakilby.com